The Science of Healthy Ageing

Unlocking the Secrets to Longevity, Vitality, and Disease Prevention

Jane Thurnell-Read

Disclaimer

While the author has used her best efforts in preparing this book, she makes no representations or warranties with respect to the accuracy or completeness of the contents of this book and specifically disclaims any implied warranties of merchantability or fitness for a particular purpose.

The information in this book is not a substitute for professional advice from your physician or other qualified healthcare provider. If appropriate, please consult with your own physician or healthcare specialist regarding the suggestions and recommendations made in this book.

Do not disregard professional medical advice or delay in seeking it because of something you have read in this book.

Spelling

US spelling and UK spelling differ in many ways.

In the UK, where I live, we write "ageing". In the US people write "aging".

In the text, I have used "ageing", except when I'm quoting a US Researcher. In these cases, I use "aging".

This also applies to other words such as fibre/fiber and analyse/analyzed, etc.

How to eat healthily: no willpower needed

Get some free help:

Healthy eating is crucial, especially when you're navigating the changes of menopause, aiming to lose weight, or simply striving to thrive as you age. Yet, wanting to eat more healthily often feels like an uphill battle.

Do you feel overwhelmed by the constant need for willpower to maintain a balanced diet? Does the struggle to eat healthily overshadow your enjoyment of life?

Imagine a life where healthy eating feels natural and effortless.

With my free eBook, "You Don't Need Willpower to Eat Healthily," you'll discover a refreshing approach to eating well. This 28-page guide offers clear explanations, enlightening insights, and practical worksheets designed to help you embrace healthier eating habits without the constant struggle.

Take the first step toward a more balanced and enjoyable life. Download your free copy today and rediscover the ease of healthy eating.

Download your free copy now and embark on a path to effortless, stress-free healthy eating:

https://www.janethurnellread.com/willpower/

Contents

1. Longevity & healthy years — 1

2. What's your reason or excuse? — 7

3. It's my age — 9

4. It's my genes — 14

5. It's too late for me now — 20

6. It'll make me so miserable — 23

7. 10 simple changes you can make now — 25

8. Diet — 31

9. Constipation — 53

10. Putting on weight as you get older — 55

11. Alcohol — 60

12. Smoking — 64

13. Exercise — 70

14. Sleep — 86

15. Dental health & gum disease — 93

16. Happiness & purpose — 96

17. Loneliness & community — 107

18. Medicines — 114

19. Supplements — 125

20. Aids & comfort   128

21. Achieving your goals   131

Books by Jane Thurnell-Read   137

About the author   138

References   140

Longevity & healthy years

D o you want to live longer? The fact that you've bought this book suggests that you do, or at least you're curious about the possibility. But most people add a rider that they only want to live longer if they stay healthy and happy. Most people wouldn't want a longer life if it meant years of chronic pain, restriction and dependency.

You want those extra years to be healthy: years when you can live life to the full. It's a crucial consideration whether extra years of life gained through increased longevity are spent in good or bad health. Scientists call them "healthy years" or "disability-free life expectancy".

What would that mean for you? Maybe you want to spend time travelling the world or learning a new sport. Maybe you want finally to master the cryptic crossword in your favourite newspaper. Perhaps you want to see your grandchildren grow up, become independent, or marry. Maybe you want to stay active in your community or engage with an important political campaign. Maybe you want healthy years just for their own sake, just for you.

All of these things need good health. They need energy, a bright mind, strength and flexibility. When I was in my fifties, I found that older people were often slow, sedentary and set in their ways. They seemed to have lost their zest for life. Many complained about being "invisible" and that nobody was interested in them or wanted to spend time with them.

At the other extreme were people like Jane Fonda. They were immaculately dressed with perfect makeup, nails and hair. They often looked very fit because they had been sporty their whole life. I couldn't identify with these women either.

I couldn't find a role model that fitted me. There were hardly any older women I aspired to be. This isn't surprising if you look at the stats for older people's health. The figures are depressing. People in the UK[1] on average stay healthy into their early sixties before they start to suffer from chronic diseases, which limit their lives in so many ways. People live on, but not in a healthy way,

Chronic diseases of old age

The US National Council on Aging[2] estimates that in the US 80% of adults 65 and older have at least one chronic condition, while 68% have two or more. These are startingly dreadful statistics. They list the ten most common conditions on their website with the percentage of over 65's who have received treatment for that condition:

- Chronic obstructive pulmonary disease (COPD) – 11%

- Alzheimer's disease and dementia – 11%

- Depression – 14%

- Heart failure – 14%

- Chronic kidney disease (CKD) -18%

- Diabetes – 27%

- Ischemic heart disease (coronary heart disease) -29%

- Arthritis – 31%

- High cholesterol – 47%

- Hypertension (high blood pressure) -58%

Looking at these figures may make you feel hopeless and disheartened.

According to the US Centers for Disease Control[3]:

"Six in ten Americans live with at least one chronic disease, like heart disease and stroke, cancer, or diabetes. These and other chronic diseases are the leading causes of death and disability in America."

The CDC goes on to say:

"We know that most chronic diseases can be prevented by eating well, being physically active, avoiding tobacco and excessive drinking, and getting regular health screenings."

The CDC estimates that over 20% of US adults over 65, who are not in care homes or hospitals are in fair or poor health. The figures for people in those institutions will be much worse.

In Canada[4] over one-third of seniors have two or more chronic diseases. Four chronic diseases (cancer, cardiovascular diseases, diabetes and chronic respiratory diseases) account for over 60% of all deaths in Canada.

In the UK the National Institute for Health and Care Research[5] has predicted that by 2035 two-thirds of adults aged over 65 are expected to be living with multiple health conditions. Seventeen percent would be living with four or more diseases.

These figures are upsetting and distressing. No wonder so many people dread getting older.

Medication use

Medicines can undoubtedly save lives or make living bearable rather than full of pain and dependence on others. But the amount of medication taken, and the number of medical errors is a cause for concern, particularly for older people who tend to take the most medication.

Many older people take a range of medications. The US Kaiser Family Foundation[6] says that 89% of adults 65 and older are currently taking prescription medicine. Medication use increases as we age. 75% of 50-64 year olds and 51% of 30-49 year olds are taking regular medication.

The statistics are even worse when you consider that many people are on more than one drug. According to the Kaiser Family Foundation, 54% of adults 65 and older are taking four or more prescription drugs compared to 32% of adults 50-64 years old. This is a truly scary statistic because drugs are tested for safety individually. They are not tested for safety or efficacy in the combinations taken by older people.

A report for England in 2017[7] found:

"... medication use [in people over 65], including both prescribed medicines and over-the-counter products has increased dramatically over the last 2 decades. The number of people taking five or more items quadrupled from 12 to 49%, while the proportion of people who did not take any medication has decreased from around 1 in 5 to 1 in 13."

I'm in my seventies. When I see my dentist, hygienist or optician, they often ask me if there is any change in my medication. They seem surprised when I say that I am not taking anything. That is because it is seen as "normal" for older people to be on long-term medication.

Inter-related health problems

You may tend to think of illnesses as separate entities. You may have two or more chronic health problems. Conventional medicine may treat these as individual problems, but this isn't always the most helpful approach.

As you will see throughout this book changing to a healthier diet will affect all your existing health problems. It can help prevent or control type 2 diabetes and improve your mental health. Exercise can improve arthritis, weight management and cancer recovery.

There are also causal relationships that are only now beginning to be understood. For example, poor dental health[8] (periodontitis) is linked with respiratory disease, rheumatoid arthritis, coronary artery disease and problems controlling blood sugar in diabetes.

If you have high blood pressure, you are probably concerned about getting heart disease or having a stroke. Interestingly, there also appears to be a relationship between high blood pressure and dementia.

In a study by the George Institute[9] (USA) over 28,000 people from 20 countries were followed for around four years. Participants had an average age of 69 and a history of high blood pressure. The study found that when people had treatment for high blood pressure they were much less likely to develop dementia.

All this is good news. Even if you are focussed on one health problem, making the recommended changes for that problem will help in other areas of your life.

Are older people sicker than they used to be?

A study from The Ohio State University[10] (USA) found that American baby boomers scored lower on a test of cognitive functioning than did members of previous generations. The research analysed data on 30,191 Americans who participated in the 1996 to 2014 Health and Retirement Survey, conducted by the University of Michigan. People over 51 years old were surveyed every two years.

As part of the study, participants completed a cognitive test in which they had to recall words they had heard earlier, count down from 100 by 7s, name objects they were shown and perform other tasks.

The UK National Institute for Health and Care Research[11] says:

"Seventeen percent [of over 65s] would be living with four or more diseases [in 2035], double the number in 2015"

It does seem highly likely that people are ageing less well. That trend is likely to continue. If I were writing this book in ten years' time, it is almost certain the figures would be even more shocking.

What's your reason or excuse?

Many people think these shocking statistics will inevitably apply to them unless they are particularly lucky or have some special genes. They believe that there is no point in taking any action because their future is beyond their control.

I want to show you that for most people this is not true. You can make significant changes to your health and well-being as you age.

But first I want to look at the most persuasive things people tell themselves so that they don't feel able to take action. They just resign themselves to the inevitable deterioration of old age.

So, what thoughts stop you from believing that you can be healthy into your old age? The most common ones are:

- It's my age. What else can I expect?

- It's my genes. Everyone in my family gets heart disease/dementia/diabetes.

- It's too late for me now. It won't make any difference what I do.

- It's too difficult. I'd rather have a short life and a happy one than do without all the things I like.

In the next chapters, I'll take each of these objections in turn and show you how you don't need to believe them.

It's my age

Many people tell me some variation of this. They believe that the health and well-being they are experiencing is directly linked to the ageing process, and that there is not much they can do about it. They may feel it's better just to accept their ill health and be at peace with that.

Your attitude to ageing

Can ageing be affected by how you think about ageing? There is intriguing research that suggests that is true.

A study[12] of 10,000 civil servants working in London found that those people who thought old age began earlier were more likely to have had a heart attack, to be suffering from heart disease or be in poor physical health generally when they were followed up six to nine years later.

The BBC website reports on this study and says:

"People who say that old age sets in at an earlier age may also be more fatalistic and less likely to seek help for medical conditions or to adopt healthier routines, believing that decline is inevitable. They may, for instance, assume that older people are frail and so deliberately start walking more slowly and taking it easy when this is exactly what they shouldn't be doing for the sake of their physical and mental health.

"They might expect to forget things due to their age, so they stop relying on their memories. It's even possible that the stress of holding negative ideas about ageing contributes to chronic inflammation and more health problems in the long term. So living up to the stereotype of an older person might increase the very problems they fear."

The American Heart Association[13] says:

"A growing body of research suggests a person's mindset – how they feel about growing old – may predict how much longer and how well they live as the years go by."

They go on to quote a US nationwide study of 14,000 adults over 50. The study found those with the highest satisfaction with aging had a 43% lower risk of dying from any cause during four years of follow-up compared to those with the lowest satisfaction. People with higher satisfaction also had a reduced risk for chronic conditions such as diabetes, stroke, cancer and heart disease, as well as better cognitive functioning. People with a more positive attitude about growing old were also more likely to engage in frequent physical activity and less likely to have trouble sleeping than their less-satisfied peers. They also were less lonely, less likely to be depressed, more optimistic and had a stronger sense of purpose.

Part of this difference seems to be that people who are more satisfied with their health are more likely to get regular checks for blood pressure and cholesterol and so on. This means problems can be spotted early and action taken. I know this should be the other way round, but the least satisfied people often fear getting tested. They may think that nothing can be done or fear invasive treatment.

Eric Kim[14], the study's senior investigator said:

"... if people believe poor health is inevitable with age, this can be a self-fulfilling prophecy that keeps them from behaviors that will help with aging"

A study in BMJ Open[15] says:

"Although ageing is generally perceived as a biologically determined process, the literature increasingly points to the importance of psychological factors in the ageing process, specifically age-related stereotypes or cognitive mind-sets. Such stereotypes reflect self-perceptions and others' perceptions about the ageing process and can have a strong influence on health and life satisfaction, specifically through self-fulfilling prophecy mechanisms."

Researchers have looked at what happens when older people are reminded about memory loss and aging before they take a memory test. They do not do as well as people who have not been reminded about these stereotypes. It's important to guard against the negativity associated with old age.

I've found that as I've got older, I've become stronger, fitter, healthier and happier. That's not what the usual stories about old age suggest. I'm constantly having to guard against the idea that the only way forward is downhill.

I post short gym videos on Instagram to inspire other older people. I want to show you that you can be strong in your sixties, seventies and beyond.

It's important to have friends who are younger than you. People in their thirties and forties don't want or need to talk about their ailments. If you surround yourself with people in their sixties and beyond, you will almost inevitably find yourself discussing illness and chronic diseases.

Be careful who you listen to. Be careful what you think. If you believe that as you get older you will get frailer and sicker, you probably will.

I'm not trying to suggest that if you think the right thoughts, you won't have any health problems in old age. If you guard your thoughts and the people you listen to, you have a better chance of living a long and healthy life.

Blue Zones

Blue zones offer overwhelming evidence that it's possible to live a healthy and long life. In Blue Zones many people lead healthy, lively and active lives into their nineties and hundreds. Living in a blue zone and following the blue zone lifestyle is protective against dementia. Research has now shown why this is so. This is not down to some special gene. It's down to their lifestyle.

The term Blue Zone first appeared in Dan Buettner's November 2005 National Geographic magazine cover story, *The Secrets of a Long Life*.

In 2004 Buettner and a group of anthropologists, demographers, epidemiologists and other researchers travelled around the world studying communities with surprisingly high percentages of centenarians. They interviewed hundreds of people who'd made it to age 100. They asked about how they lived. Then the scientists looked at the data to understand what these thriving elderly people had in common.

The five Blue Zones are Ikari in Greece, Okinawa in Japan, Ogliastra Region in Sardinia, Loma Linda in USA and Nicoya Peninsula in Costa Rica. These are very specific communities – it's not the whole of the island of Sardinia or the whole of California. It's a special community.

So, what is special about these communities? Researchers have come up with recommendations based on the lives of these exceptional people:

- Stop eating when your stomach is 80 % full to avoid weight gain.

- Eat the smallest meal of the day in the late afternoon or evening.

- Eat mostly plants, especially beans.

- Eat meat rarely, in small portions of 85 to 113 gr (3 to 4 ounces). Blue Zoners eat portions this size just five times a month, on average.

- Drink alcohol moderately and regularly, just 1-2 glasses a day. (If you have problems moderating your alcohol consumption, this is of course not advisable.)

- Be part of a community with a sense of purpose. For many Blue Zone inhabitants, this was strong shared religious beliefs. (There are other ways that people who lack religious beliefs can develop a sense of community and shared purpose, and these may be equally effective.)

The important message from Blue Zone communities is that decline, frailty, dementia and chronic illnesses aren't inevitable as you age. It can be different if you incorporate at least some of these changes in your own life.

The Blue Zones are messages of hope for the rest of us as we contemplate the years ahead.

The United Nations also offers a message of hope. Many older people suffer from the chronic diseases associated with old age (heart problems, diabetes, respiratory problems, arthritis and so on). Many people assume this is normal ageing, but the United Nations website[16] says:

"The combination of four healthy lifestyle factors - maintaining a healthy weight, exercising regularly, following a healthy diet, and not smoking - seem to be associated with as much as an 80 per cent reduction in the risk of developing the most common and deadly chronic diseases. "

All this tells us that it may seem normal to have one or more chronic illnesses as you get older, but it definitely doesn't have to be. A healthy lifestyle can pay dividends.

You may feel that you are likely to suffer from cancer, as you get older. The statistics in most countries are truly horrendous. In the UK, for example, Cancer Research UK [17]says that 1 in 2 of us will develop cancer during our lifetime. There are childhood cancers, but the vast majority of cancer sufferers are older people. Cancer Research UK goes on to say that around 4 in 10 UK cancer cases every year could be prevented. OK, we'd all like that figure to be all cancers can be prevented, but even 4 in 10 is a lot.

When the charity talks about preventable cancers, it's not talking here about preventable through medical intervention. It means lifestyle changes. The lifestyle changes it is advocating are also the lifestyle changes that will help you live longer.

I hope this information has inspired you to believe that you can stay well into old age. It's not just simply a matter of luck.

It's my genes

M any people seem to think that the reason I'm fit and well is because of my genes. I am fit and healthy partly because of my genes, but is also down to the way I eat, the amount of exercise I take, and my interest and participation in life. It's partly down to luck. I've had many great things happen in my life. But genes and luck don't explain everything about my health and well-being. Genes and luck don't explain everything about your level of health and well-being.

Some people do have an increased risk of some illnesses (such as some cancers, type 2 diabetes and frontotemporal dementia) because they have an inherited gene fault. Even in these situations, the development of that specific illness may not be inevitable. It may be that there are things you can do to delay the onset.

Genes and disease risks

Researchers at the University of Alberta (Canada) reviewed all the main studies over the last 20 years examining the relationships between common gene mutations and different diseases and conditions. They concluded[18]:

"In most cases, your genes have less than five per cent to do with your risk of developing a particular disease."

They go on to say:

"It is becoming increasingly clear that the risks for getting most diseases arise from your metabolism, your environment, your lifestyle, or your exposure to various kinds of nutrients, chemicals, bacteria, or viruses."

The website Genes In Life[19] says:

"You can't change your genes, but you can change your behavior. There are steps you can take to prevent disease, lower your risk, and find problems early when most treatments work best."

Professor Dean Ornish is the president and founder of the non-profit Preventive Medicine Research Institute in Sausalito, California (USA). He says:

"Your genes are not your fate... if you change your lifestyle, you change your genes."

Your epigenome

The epigenome refers to a set of chemical modifications that can occur on your DNA and its surrounding proteins, without actually changing the underlying genetic code. You still have the same genes, but the epigenome turns the gene on or off, and so influences various aspects of your health.

While your DNA provides the blueprint for your body's structure and function, the epigenome can act as a kind of "interpreter," helping to translate your genetic information into actual traits and behaviours. These modifications can be influenced by a variety of factors, including your environment, diet, stress levels, and even your experiences and behaviours.

A study from Washington State University[20] (USA) followed 70 pairs of identical twins from 2012 to 2019. It found that the more physically active siblings had lower signs of metabolic disease, measured by waist size and body mass index. This also correlated with differences in their epigenomes. The more active twins had epigenetic marks linked to lowered metabolic syndrome, reducing the risk of heart disease, stroke and type 2 diabetes.

Because the twins were identical and had the same genes this is important evidence that a healthy lifestyle influences health outcomes. If genetics and DNA sequence were the only drivers for biology, then essentially twins should have the same diseases. But they don't necessarily.

Genes and old age

People often get sicker as they grow older, but research from Gil McVean[21] of the University of Oxford (UK) and colleagues finds that the impact of a person's genes on their risk of getting sick actually wanes with age. McVean says:

"Our work shows that the way in which genetics affects your risk of getting a disease change throughout life. For many diseases, genetic factors are most important in determining whether you will get a disease early in life, while - as you age - other factors come to dominate risk."

This understanding has also been supported by work from researchers[22] at UC Berkeley (USA). They found:

" ... while our individual genetic makeup can help predict gene expression when we are younger, it is less useful in predicting which genes are ramped up or down when we're older [more than 55 years old] ... Identical twins, for example, have the same set of genes, but as they age, their gene expression profiles diverge, meaning that twins can age much differently from each other."

Isn't that a cheering thought? Your genes will continue to have less and less influence on your health as you age. It's more and more down to you. I hope this is an exciting thought. You can change your life for the better. That may be a scary thought, but I aim to help you. In this book, you'll find practical tools and strategies you can use to make that a reality. I want you to see this as a time of opportunity.

Genes and cancer

Cancer Research UK[23] says:

"As well as a gene fault, many other factors need to be in place for a cancer to develop. Because the other factors are not always in place, the cancer may seem to skip a generation. A parent may have the gene and not develop cancer but their child who inherits the same gene does develop cancer."

The World Cancer Research Fund[24] says:

"Only about 5-10% of all cancer cases result from specific inherited genes ... People who inherit gene mutations ... have a higher than average risk of developing some types of cancer, though it doesn't mean they will definitely get cancer."

The website goes on to say:

"You can lower your risk of developing many types of cancer by not smoking, followed by maintaining a healthy weight through keeping active and eating a healthy diet."

A study from the American Association for Cancer Research[25] found that:

"Healthy lifestyle factors such as abstinence from smoking and drinking, low body mass index, and exercise correlated with decreased cancer incidence, even in individuals with a high genetic risk."

A study from the Vanderbilt University Medical Center[26] (USA) found that:

"People with a high polygenic risk score for colorectal cancer could benefit more at preventing the disease by leading healthy lifestyles than those at lower genetic risk.

"In the analysis, lifestyle scores of unhealthy, intermediate and healthy were determined according to waist-to-hip ratio, physical activity, sedentary time, processed and red meat intake, vegetable and fruit intake, alcohol consumption and tobacco use."

Genes and dementia

A study published in the journal Alzheimer's & Dementia[27] looked at people who carried a gene linked to frontotemporal lobar degeneration (FTLD), which is a type of dementia. Subjects with the gene who engaged in active cognitive and physical lifestyles had a 55% slower rate of cognitive decline than patients who weren't active in this way. This, of course, doesn't mean that they weren't affected by the gene they carried. It does mean that the deterioration was delayed significantly. The idea that if you "have a gene for something bad" you will necessarily have no control over what happens to you is far from the truth.

Genes and type 2 diabetes

Genes can affect the likelihood of you getting type 2 diabetes. So can your lifestyle, particularly your diet. Researchers[28] analysed data from over 35,000 men and women, who had participated in three long-term studies. They concluded that a healthy diet is associated with lower diabetes risk across all levels of genetic risk. Even if you have a high risk of developing type 2 diabetes, eating a healthy diet will reduce that risk.

Longevity and early death

In 2012 researchers from the University of San Diego[29] (USA) began measuring the physical activity of 5,446 women in the United States who were 63 and older. They followed them through until 2020. The study found that higher levels of light physical activity and moderate-to-vigorous physical activity were associated with a lower risk of death. Higher sedentary time was associated with a higher risk of mortality. These associations were consistent among women regardless of their genetic predisposition for longevity.

Senior author, Assistant Professor Aladdin H. Shadyab says:

"Our study showed that, even if you aren't likely to live long based on your genes, you can still extend your lifespan by engaging in positive lifestyle behaviors such as regular exercise and sitting less. Conversely, even if your genes predispose you to a long life, remaining physically active is still important to achieve longevity."

It's too late for me now

Many people in their fifties or sixties feel too old to turn their health around. They believe that there is no point in trying because it won't make any difference. Research emphatically says that is not true. In this book there are examples of research showing people can turn round diabetes, pain, frailty and much more. They can even reduce their biological age.

Chronological age is the age calculated from your birth certificate. Biological age is also called physiological age. It reflects how your body is ageing and how your systems are functioning. While you can do nothing about your chronological age, research shows you can do something about your biological age.

Researchers[30] published details of a study in the academic journal Aging in 2021 on whether lifestyle interventions can change your biological age.

43 healthy adult males between the ages of 50-72 took part in an 8-week study. The treatment group followed a programme that included diet, sleep, exercise and relaxation guidance, and supplements (probiotics and phytonutrients). The control group received no intervention. The participants' biological age was established by analysing saliva samples. The treatment group experienced an average 1.96 years decrease in biological age by the end of the programme compared to the same individuals at the beginning. This was after an intervention that only lasted eight weeks.

This is a small study only involving men. There isn't any information on the ethnicity of the participants, so it clear that more work needs to be done in this area. Even so, this confirms what the research on individual diseases shows: you can become younger if you adopt the right lifestyle.

Johns Hopkins-led Multi-Ethnic Study of Atherosclerosis[31] tracked more than 6,000 people ages 44 to 84 for over seven years. They found that those who made lifestyle changes such as quitting smoking, following a Mediterranean-style diet, getting regular exercise and maintaining a healthy weight decreased their risk of death in that time by 80 percent.

A study involving 15,708 participants published in the American Journal of Medicine[32] concluded:

"People who newly adopt a healthy lifestyle in middle-age experience a prompt benefit of lower rates of cardiovascular disease and mortality."

A study by the European Society of Cardiology[33] found that it is never too late to get active. The study followed 30,000 people with an average age of 62. They were followed on average for 7 years.

The researchers examined the risks of all-cause death and death from cardiovascular disease. Compared to patients who were inactive over that time, the risk of all-cause death was 50% lower in those who were active over that time, 45% lower in those who were inactive but became active, and 20% lower in those who had been active but became inactive.

There's an interesting study[34] that has shown that men with prostate cancer can significantly reduce the chances of the disease worsening by eating more fruits, vegetables, nuts and olive oil. The study of 2000 men with prostate cancer showed that making these changes can lead to a nearly 50% reduction in the risk of prostate cancer progression.

Senior author Professor Stacey A. Kenfield said:

"Making small changes in one's diet each day is beneficial. ... Greater consumption of plant-based food after a prostate cancer diagnosis has also recently been associated with better quality of life, including sexual function, urinary function and vitality, so it's a win-win on both levels."

This research does show it's never too late to make the lifestyle changes that can help you live longer and better.

Yet it's clear the younger you start the lifestyle changes the earlier you will see the results. A study published in PLOS Medicine in 2022 based on the results of several research projects concluded:

"... prolonged dietary changes at age 20 years would give about 48% higher gain in LE [life expectancy] as changes starting from age 60 years, and 3 times the gains when compared with changes starting at age 80 years ... Similar findings were seen for China and the United States."

This doesn't mean you are too old to change, even if you are 80 years old. It just means you'll experience fewer benefits than younger people would. The researchers developed a website[35] where you can enter your age and the amount of each category of food you eat each day and see the effect it has on your life expectancy. The food groups are whole grains, fruits, vegetables, nuts, legumes, fish, eggs, milk/dairy, refined grains, red meat, processed meat, and sugar-sweetened beverages. You can compare your life expectancy on your current diet with your life expectancy if you increased, decreased or eliminated a particular food group.

Remember this isn't so much about looking younger, though that will probably happen. It's not just about preventing your own death. It's about functioning as though you are younger. If you are functioning younger, you are likely to experience less pain, more energy and need less medication. You are likely to experience more healthy years.

It'll make me so miserable

The changes I describe in this book demand you make changes to your lifestyle. You may contemplate that idea with a sinking heart.

Surely a short, but happy life is better than one of deprivation and exercise. This is a wrong conclusion on two counts.

Firstly, most people don't have a wonderful, happy, indulgent life and then drop dead. That's just not how your body works.

Most older people suffer from the chronic diseases associated with old age. You may not have a short life. Many older people have ten or more years of breathlessness, pain, anxiety and illness. Most older people become frailer and more dependent on others for even the most intimate personal tasks. That's not a short and happy life.

Secondly, research shows categorically that eating well is likely to increase your happiness – food and mood are inextricably linked. Research has shown without a shadow of a doubt that exercise, even irregular exercise, can lead you to feel more optimistic and energetic. Sleep research shows that getting enough sleep is fundamental to your well-being and your ability to function in the day-to-day world. Giving up smoking will save you money and is likely to improve your mental health too. Reducing your alcohol consumption will also save you money, and lead to better mental health. These changes may make you unhappy in the short run, but long-term you are likely to end up happier.

The changes I set out in this book will give you the best chance of living a happy and healthy life. Ask yourself, if you carry on as you are, how likely is it that you will be happy and healthy in the future?

Of course, some people have a very unhealthy lifestyle but live to be fit and well into their eighties and beyond. You may know some of these people. But they are a very, very small minority. If you are relying on being one of these people, you are taking a very big gamble with the rest of your life.

10 simple changes you can make now

I want to start with some easy, simple changes you can start with right now. Each one is backed by research about what works. Don't try all ten at the same time. Read through them all and find the one that is easiest to implement. Start with that. Once it's part of your everyday life add another one.

Walk 3800 steps

Have you read that you should walk 10,000 steps a day? If you hardly walk anywhere, the idea of doing 10,000 steps each day may be appalling. But don't despair, here's some research to inspire you. Researchers from the University of Sydney[36] (Australia) found that 3,800 steps a day can cut your risk of dementia by 25 percent.

Even that many steps may be too much for you initially. If it is, make a start. Set your sights on walking every day and adding more steps each day. Could you add an extra 100 steps each day until you can celebrate your first milestone – 3,800 steps a day? If that's too much, aim to add 100 steps every few days or even once a week. The important thing is that you do this and make consistent progress from the level you started at.

The same researchers found that achieving 10,000 steps a day lowered the risk of dementia, heart disease, cancer and death. When you're comfortable walking

3,800 steps a day, know that you can get even more benefits by increasing the number of steps you take.

Add herbs and spices to your diet

Researchers from Penn University[37] (USA) analysed the impact of adding blends of herbs and spices to the controlled diets of participants at risk for cardiovascular disease. The blend used was cinnamon, ginger, cumin, turmeric, rosemary, oregano, basil and thyme. The team examined three doses:

- about 1/8 teaspoon per day

- a little more than 3/4 teaspoon per day

- 1.5 teaspoon per day.

At the end of four weeks, participants showed an increased gut bacteria diversity, particularly with the medium and high doses of herbs and spices. Research shows categorically that having a lot of different gut bacteria is beneficial for your health.

Professor Penny M. Kris-Etherton

"It's such a simple thing that people can do. The average American diet is far from ideal, so I think everyone could benefit by adding herbs and spices. It's also a way of decreasing sodium in your diet by flavoring foods in a way that makes them palatable and, in fact, delicious! Taste is really a top criterion for why people choose the foods they do."

So help your gut bacteria and reduce your salt intake by adding this spice combination to your food every day.

Drink 500 ml of water before meals

Elizabeth A Dennis and colleagues[38] conducted an experiment in which half the participants drank 500 ml (1.06 US pints) of water before meals. After 12 weeks weight loss was around 2 kg (4.4 lb) greater in the water group than in the non-water group. This was a 44% greater decline in weight over the 12 weeks for participants who drank water before meals.

All the participants were middle-aged and older adults and followed a low-calorie diet for 12 weeks. There is every reason to think this would apply whatever your age and whether or not you are reducing your calories.

Drinking a glass of water before each meal is an easy thing to do, isn't it?

Eat almonds every day

Gut health is so important. It can affect so many other aspects of your health, so it's great to know that eating almonds every day may improve your gut health. Researchers from the University of London[39] recruited 87 healthy adults who were already eating less than the recommended amount of dietary fibre and who snacked on typical unhealthy snacks (e.g. chocolate, crisps). Participants were split into three groups:

- Group 1 changed their snacks to 56 g (just under 2 ounces) of whole almonds a day

- Group 2 ate 56 g of ground almonds a day

- Group 3, the control group, ate energy-matched muffins as a control

The trial lasted four weeks. Researchers found that butyrate was significantly higher among almond eaters compared to those who consumed the muffin. You probably don't know what this means, so let me explain.

Butyrate is a short-chain fatty acid that is the main source of fuel for the cells lining the colon. When these cells function effectively, it provides an ideal condition for gut microbes to flourish, for the gut wall to be strong (not leaky or inflamed) and for nutrients to be absorbed. An unhealthy gut lining may have large cracks or holes, allowing partially digested food, toxins, and bugs to penetrate the tissues beneath it. This may trigger inflammation and changes in the gut flora (normal bacteria) that could lead to problems within the digestive tract and beyond.

You can now forget all that explanation. Just remember that a daily snack of almonds (56 g or 2 ounces) will benefit your health if you don't normally eat much fibre and many healthy snacks. If you're not used to eating nuts, you may want to start with a smaller amount and chew them well.

Control your snacking

Keep healthy snacks in clear containers at the front of the fridge or cupboard. Put unhealthy snacks at the back of the cupboard or fridge. Put them in plain dark containers. Simple changes like this can mean that you eat fewer unhealthy snacks.

Snack from a plate, not the packet -- it is easy to feel you should finish the packet. Put what you want on a plate and put the rest of the pack out of sight.

Write a gratitude letter

Research by Martin E. P. Seligman found that volunteers who wrote and presented a letter of gratitude to someone they had never properly thanked were significantly happier and less depressed three months later. He doesn't say how the person receiving the letter was, but they may have been happier too. Try it yourself.

Eat peanuts

Replace one high carbohydrate snack (such as cake or cookies or crisps/chips) with 28 grams (approximately 1 ounce) of peanuts every day. Don't choose salted peanuts, as too much salt can raise your blood pressure. Researchers at Penn University[40] (USA) found that eating peanuts in this way increased the abundance of a group of bacteria linked to healthy liver metabolism and immune function.

Take a walking break

Many people sit more as they get older or have sedentary jobs. Sitting for long periods of time has been linked to an increased risk of cardiovascular disease and early death. But a study by Columbia University (USA) exercise physiologists[41] found that just five minutes of walking every half hour during periods of prolonged sitting can offset some of the most harmful effects.

Doing this significantly lowered both blood sugar and blood pressure. In addition, this walking regimen had a dramatic effect on how the participants responded to large meals, reducing blood sugar spikes by 58% compared with sitting all day. The researchers also found it led to significant decreases in fatigue and significant improvements in mood.

Even taking a walking break every 30 minutes for one minute provided modest benefits for blood sugar levels throughout the day. So make a start with that, but aim to walk for 5 minutes every 30 minutes as soon as possible.

Do vigorous exercise for around a minute

A study from the University of Sydney (Australia)[42] found that one-minute bursts of activity during daily tasks could prolong your life. These short bursts of vigorous activity are known as VILPA:

"VILPA is the very short bouts of vigorous activity (up to one to two minutes) we do with gusto each day, like running for the bus, bursts of power walking while doing errands or playing high-energy games with the kids."

The researchers found that just three to four one-minute bouts of VILPA every day is associated with up to 40 percent reduction in all-cause and cancer-related mortality, and up to a 49 percent reduction in death related to cardiovascular disease. They studied 100,000 people, which gives huge credibility to their findings.

You can surely do 3-4 minutes of exercise every day no matter how busy you are. But remember it needs to be vigorous exercise, although for a very short period of time.

Professor Emmanuel Stamakakis says:

"It requires no time commitment, no preparation, no club memberships, no special skills. It simply involves stepping up the pace while walking or doing the housework with a bit more energy. "

Take a bath before bed

Researchers from the University of Texas (USA)[43] found that bathing 1-2 hours before bedtime in water of about 104-109 degrees Fahrenheit (40 - 43 degrees Celsius) can significantly improve your sleep.

Diet

In an earlier chapter I quoted from the United Nations website[44] that four lifestyle changes could result in an 80% reduction in the chronic diseases associated with old age. Eating a healthy diet is one of these.

Following a healthy diet can avoid or delay the start of some chronic illnesses. A healthy diet can also help with the severity of many diseases. Even if you've never had a healthy diet, it is not too late to start now.

Longevity diet and fasting

Professor Valter Longo and colleagues from the University of Southern California[45] reviewed hundreds of studies on nutrition, diseases and longevity in laboratory animals and humans. They combined them with their own studies on nutrition and aging. They concluded that the key characteristics of the optimal diet appear to be moderate to high carbohydrate intake from non-refined sources, low but sufficient protein from largely plant-based sources, and enough plant-based fats to provide about 30 percent of energy needs.

Professor Longo described what eating for longevity could look like in real life:

"Lots of legumes, whole grains, and vegetables; some fish; no red meat or processed meat and very low white meat; low sugar and refined grains; good levels of nuts and olive oil, and some dark chocolate."

He also offers advice on meal timing. Ideally, the day's meals would all occur within a window of 11-12 hours, allowing for a daily period of fasting. So, for example, if you normally eat your breakfast at 8 am you should have finished eating your evening meal before 8 pm. This may be very easy for you to do. You may already be doing it without realising that you were creating a daily period of fasting.

If you're used to having a late supper, or eating something just before you go to bed, you will need to make some changes. Of course, you could eat something late in the evening, but then you would need to wait until late morning the next day before eating anything. In general, eating within 3 hours of your bedtime is not recommended[46]. It can disturb sleep and some researchers[47] say it can also lead to weight gain.

Professor Longo also advocates a 5-day cycle of a fasting or fasting-mimicking diet every 3-4 months, as it may help reduce insulin resistance, lower blood pressure and other risk factors for individuals who are most at risk of chronic diseases.

A fasting-mimicking diet is a type of diet that is designed to mimic the effects of a water-only fast while still allowing you to consume some food. It usually involves drastically reducing calorie intake for a short period of time, while still consuming small amounts of nutrient-dense foods.

Typically, a fasting-mimicking diet involves consuming around 500-800 calories per day, with a focus on nutrient-dense, whole foods such as vegetables, nuts, and healthy fats. You would do this for 5 days every 3-4 months. While this is likely to be safe and beneficial for most people, you may want to consult your medical adviser if you already have health problems.

Mediterranean diet

The traditional Mediterranean diet is eaten by people in the countries bordering the Mediterranean, such as Greece and Italy. Scientists became interested in looking at the diet in more detail when it was noticed that heart disease and stroke were less common in these countries than in the USA and UK.

In these countries, people traditionally eat predominantly plant-based foods, such as grains, vegetables, legumes/beans, fruits, nuts, seeds, herbs and spices. Olive oil is the main source of added fat. Wine is also drunk by many people, but only in moderation. Researchers say alcohol is not an essential part of a healthy Mediterranean diet.

Fish, seafood, dairy and poultry are eaten in moderation. Red meat and sweets are eaten only occasionally. The diet contains very little ultra-processed foods bought ready-made from supermarkets and fast-food outlets.

This diet is, of course, very similar to the diet for longevity discussed earlier. People who follow this diet[48] have:

- longer lives

- fewer cardiovascular problems, including heart disease and stroke

- less obesity, hypertension, metabolic syndrome, and dyslipidaemia

- lower rates of incident diabetes, and better glycaemic control if they are a diabetic compared to control diets

- less age-related cognitive dysfunction and lower incidence of neurodegenerative disorders, particularly Alzheimer's disease

In addition, this diet has much less environmental impact than the standard Western diet.

Many people feel they can follow the Mediterranean diet without too much difficulty. Could you? Focus on what you can (and should eat) rather than what you need to moderate or eliminate. This doesn't mean you can never eat birthday cake or chicken nuggets again. It does mean that the majority of your diet is plant-based. Because many of the benefits of a Mediterranean diet are long-term, it may take a while before you are aware of them. Be patient and know that you are feeding your body in the best way possible.

More plant foods

Over 400,000 people were followed in the USA from 1995 to 2011[49]. The median age was just over 62 years old. The researchers found that replacing 3% energy from animal protein with plant protein decreased the risk of dying by 10% in both men and women.

This seems very doable – change 3% of your calories from animal protein (meat, fish, dairy, eggs, and so on) for the same quantity of plant protein (nuts, seeds, legumes, tofu etc.) You can do that, can't you?

Eat the rainbow

So far, I've talked about the benefits of focussing on a diet with lots of vegetables and fruit. You will be doing your body even more favours if you vary the colour of the vegetables and fruits you eat. People call this eating the rainbow.

Colourful fruit and vegetables look good on the plate. But there are other more important reasons to make sure you eat colourful meals.

Fruit and vegetables contain phytonutrients (also known as phytochemicals). They help the plants resist pests and the harmful effects of radiation and UV rays. But they are also extremely important for your health. Phytochemicals are not essential nutrients (like vitamins and minerals are) but are substances in food that have been found to enhance health. For example, they reduce the risk of cardiovascular disease, certain cancers, dementia and age-related blindness.

At least 900 different phytonutrients have been identified. Different fruits and vegetables contain different phytonutrients. Different phytonutrients benefit your health in different ways.

For example, some phytonutrient molecules are too big to go through the gut wall, so they work in the gut itself. Some are water-soluble so can go where the fat-soluble ones can't. Some work on the surface of cells and some work inside cells. You want a range of phytonutrients, so that they will work everywhere in your body to help prevent damage and decay.

A study[50] followed almost 70,000 people over 20 years. Participants completed questionnaires from time to time about what they ate and also about their cognitive abilities (memory etc.) After adjusting for factors like age and total caloric intake, people who consumed more flavonoids in their diets reported lower risk of cognitive decline. The group of highest flavonoid consumers had 20% less risk of self-reported cognitive decline than the people in the lowest group. The researchers found that orange fruit and vegetables were particularly effective.

So, you need to eat a range of different fruit and vegetables to ensure you get the biggest range of phytonutrients you can. Fortunately, some of the phytochemicals give fruit and vegetables their colour. This explains why eating colourful food is healthy. By eating a range of colours (the rainbow) you are automatically eating a range of phytochemicals.

The American Heart Association[51] agrees that you need to eat the rainbow:

"The best way to get all of the vitamins, minerals and nutrients you need is to eat a variety of colorful fruits and veggies. Add color to your plate each day with the five main color groups.

- Red & Pink foods such as beets, cherries, radicchio, red peppers, red apples.

- Blue & Purple foods include blackberries, blueberries, dates, eggplants (aubergine) and grapes.

- Yellow & Orange foods include butternut squash, oranges, corn, apricots, orange peppers and nectarines.

- White foods include bananas, cauliflower, garlic, potatoes and mush-
  rooms.

- Green foods include asparagus, avocados, bok choy, broccoli, celery
  and green onions."

Eat 30 different fruits/veggies a week

So far we've looked at eating more plants with a focus on eating a range of
colours for their phytochemical benefits. But eating a variety of different plants
has a benefit for your gut microbiome. Researchers at the American Gut Project
found that people who ate more than 30 different plant foods each week had a
more diverse gut microbiome compared with those who ate 10 or fewer.

The research also showed that people who achieved the 30 varieties also had
more bacteria that produce something called short-chain fatty acids. These fatty
acids have been shown to reduce your risk of bowel cancer.

A diverse gut microbiome is associated with better overall health. It's good
for your immune system and reduces your risk of common chronic diseases such
as type 2 diabetes and heart disease.

The World Cancer Research Fund[52] has an excellent summary on their
website of what this means in practice:

- "Fruit and vegetables are obviously plant foods: each variety can count
  as one – so a cos lettuce is different from watercress, rocket(arugula)
  and iceberg.

- "Legumes: beans, such as black, cannellini or kidney, chickpeas, and
  lentils. Each type counts as one.

- "Grains: oats, buckwheat, millet, wheat, brown rice, wholemeal pasta
  and quinoa. White pasta and rice aren't included, because the industrial processes used to remove the wholegrains strip them of many of

their nutritional benefits.

- "Nuts and seeds: almonds, hazelnuts, sunflower seeds, pumpkin seeds, cashews and so on. Again each type counts as one.

- "Herbs and spices: because the quantities you eat tend to be fairly small, each is only counted as one-quarter."

Remember that the foods also count if they are frozen or canned. Salads, soups and stir-fries can add a lot of variety easily. Many of us eat similar food on most days. If you do this your gut microbiome will suffer and, in the long term, so will your health. Make a conscious decision when shopping to buy a bigger variety of fruit and vegetables. Be adventurous and try new ones. Hopefully, you will find something you really like.

Eating 30 different plants and eating the rainbow work well together. In doing both you are really increasing your chances of living healthily and well into your old age.

Superfoods

Sadly, many people are searching for miracle foods to help them live a long and healthy life. There are lots of blogs and influencer posts praising one particular food – blueberries or salmon, for example - as the key to longevity.

Of course, this is an appealing idea. It would be nice to think that I can eat whatever I like, provided I have a particular superfood every day. But this is clearly a fantasy idea. Dr Shireen Kassam[53], founder of Plant Based Health Professionals says:

"It is more useful to consider healthy diet patterns rather than individual foods that promote longevity."

You need to eat a whole range of healthy foods and avoid or limit a whole range of unhealthy foods in order to be healthy and well. Chasing after one or two superfoods that will transform your life is sadly not a good strategy for a long and healthy life.

Fats and fatty food

A small amount of fat is an essential part of a healthy, balanced diet. Fat is a source of essential fatty acids, which your body needs but cannot make itself. Fat also helps your body absorb vitamins A, D and E. These vitamins are fat-soluble, which means they can only be absorbed with the help of fats.

Helpguide.org[54] says:

"Since fat is an important part of a healthy diet, rather than adopting a low-fat diet, it's more important to focus on eating more beneficial "good" fats and limiting harmful "bad" fats."

Trans fats are very bad fats. Saturated fats are bad fats. Unsaturated fats are good fats.

Trans fats are created while cooking, particularly at high temperatures. Many processed foods have high levels of transfats: cookies, cakes, pastries, and dough-nuts, French fries, crisps (chips), margarine, non-dairy creamers, fried chicken, burgers and other fried food. Transfats are known to have negative impacts on health. For example, trans fats have been shown to increase levels of "bad" LDL cholesterol while decreasing levels of "good" HDL cholesterol, leading to an increased risk of heart disease and stroke.

Saturated fat comes from many different sources, including meat, chicken, butter, dairy products and palm and coconut oil. This advice about reduc-ing saturated fats echoes the recommendation from longevity diets and the Mediterranean diet: reduce meat, dairy and processed foods.

Monounsaturated fats (MUFAs) include olive oil, avocado oil, peanut oil, rapeseed (canola) oil, sesame oil, sunflower oil, almond oil and hazelnut oil. MUFAs have been associated with improving insulin sensitivity, reducing the risk of heart disease and stroke, and reducing inflammation.

Polyunsaturated fats (PUFAs) include flaxseed oil, walnut oil, soyabean oil, corn oil, sunflower oil and fatty fish oil. These have also been shown to be associated with better heart health and less inflammation, as well as better cognitive health. But too high an intake has been associated with an increase in chronic diseases.

You may well often cook with oil, so you need to know which oils you should use. Some oils are better suited to high-temperature cooking than others. That's because some oils change structurally when they're heated, turning into unhealthy substances.

Oils[55] with high smoke-points are good for high-heat frying and stir-frying. These include peanut, sesame and soybean. Oils with moderately high smoke points are good for sauteing over medium-high heat. These include avocado, corn, rapeseed (also called canola) and olive oil.

You may now be feeling overwhelmed with all this information about fats, so let me try and simplify it for you in terms of what you need to do:

- Reduce trans fats by reducing the amount of processed baked goods and fried food you eat.

- Reduce the amount of saturated fat in your diet by reducing meat and dairy.

- Cook with peanut oil or sesame or soyabean oil when cooking at high temperatures.

- Cook with corn, olive or rapeseed (canola) oil when sauteing.

- Use olive oil or peanut oil on your salads and veggies.

- Include some polyunsaturated oil in your diet either as a food or as an oil – walnuts, sunflowers and fatty fish.

- Remember that oils are high in calories, so be careful of quantities if you are watching your weight.

- Remember that unsaturated fats are essential for your health, and you should not try to exclude all fats from your diet.

This may still seem overwhelming. If it is, take just one of these (the easiest one) and apply that in your life. Then add the others over time.

Nuts and seeds

Eating nuts and seeds used to be discouraged on the grounds that they were very high calorie snacks. Tufts University (USA) Health & Nutrition Letter[56] says:

"Nuts and seeds are a rich source of plant protein, have plenty of dietary fiber, and are high in heart-healthy mono-and polyunsaturated fats (including plant omega-3 fatty acids) and low in saturated fats. They also contain many vitamins and minerals (such as vitamin E, magnesium, phosphorus, copper, and manganese) and a collection of plant chemicals with potential antioxidant and anti-inflammatory properties."

The general recommendation is to have a small handful of nuts and seeds every day. If you tend to eat unhealthy snacks, replacing them with a handful of nuts or seeds will bring even more benefit.

Ultra-processed food

Ultra-processed foods include packaged baked goods, sugary cereals, many snacks, fizzy drinks, and ready-to-eat or heat products. They often contain high levels of added sugar, fat, and/or salt. They usually contain chemicals such as emulsifiers and stabilisers that prolong shelf-life. They usually lack vitamins and fibre and contain no raw ingredients.

All this makes them super tasty and tempting to buy. Ultra-processed foods usually mean you don't need to spend much time and energy on food preparation. Shops and supermarkets also find ultra-processed food easy to stock, unlike fresh fruit and vegetables, which are perishable.

Richard Hoffman[57] from the University of Hertfordshire (UK) writes:

"In countries such as the UK, US and Canada, ultra-processed foods now account for 50% or more of calories consumed. This is concerning, given that these foods have been linked to a number of different health conditions, including a greater risk of obesity and various chronic diseases such as cardiovascular disease and dementia."

Not having a diet with a high proportion of ultra-processed food takes commitment and time. But the rewards for this are likely to be a healthier and happier you.

A study published in the medical journal BMJ[58] followed 105,159 French adults with an average age of 43 years for 10 years. The researchers found an absolute 10% increase in the proportion of ultra-processed food in the diet was associated with significantly higher rates of overall cardiovascular disease (12%), coronary heart disease (13%), and cerebrovascular disease (11%).

In contrast, the researchers also found a significant association between unprocessed or minimally processed foods and lower risks of all reported diseases.

Another study also published in the BMJ[59] was based on nearly 20,000 Spanish university graduates with an average age of 38. They were followed for an average of 10 years. Results showed that higher consumption of ultra-processed foods (more than 4 servings per day) was associated with a 62% increased risk of all-cause mortality compared with lower consumption (less than 2 servings per day).

Both these studies suggest a link between consumption of ultra-processed food and mortality, but it can't be said conclusively that one causes the other. There has been research that suggests what mechanisms could cause an increase in mortality from ultra-processed food consumption.

Some food additives common in ultra-processed foods (such as emulsifiers and artificial sweeteners) also increase inflammation in the gut by causing changes to the gut microbiome. A healthy gut microbiome is important for your health and well-being, so this is concerning.

All of this suggests that minimising your intake of ultra-processed foods is an extremely important strategy for healthy ageing. It means you will need to resist the blandishments of advertising and supermarkets but remember these companies do not have your interests at heart. They just want you to buy more of these products to help them as a company succeed.

A study published in the journal Public Health Nutrition[60] found that over half of the ultra-processed foods they looked at contained a nutritional claim on their packaging and a quarter had a health claim. This sort of messaging can lull you into a belief that you are making a healthy choice, but fundamentally the evidence says that ultra-processed food is bad for you, regardless of what claims the manufacturer makes.

This is probably one of the best things you can do for yourself: reduce the amount of ultra-processed food you eat on a regular basis.

Salt

Many people use more salt on their food as they get older. Carolyn Ross[61] of Washington State University (USA) says:

"... the ability to taste and smell is known to weaken with age, and weaker perception of salty flavors may induce people to season their food with excessive salt, which may increase their risk of cardiovascular disease."

According to WHO[62] most people (not just older people) consume too much salt. On average it's 9–12 grams per day, or around twice the recommended maximum level of intake. An estimated 2.5 million deaths could be prevented each year if global salt consumption were reduced to the recommended level.

Salt intake of less than 5 grams per day for adults helps to reduce blood pressure and risk of cardiovascular disease, stroke and coronary heart attack. 5 grams is just under a teaspoon of salt but remember this is salt from all sources including breakfast cereals, processed foods, bread and processed meals. It's not just about the salt you add from a salt-shaker.

The American Heart Association[63] estimates that 75% or more of daily sodium intake in the USA is from processed/packaged foods and restaurant foods. Yet another reason to reduce your intake of processed food.

The Queensland Government health website[64] (Australia) gives this advice for choosing processed food: "Try to aim for items that have less than 120mg of sodium per 100 grams of the food."

WHO recommends that you reduce your salt intake at home by:

- not adding salt during the preparation of food

- not having a salt-shaker on the table

- limiting the consumption of salty snacks

- choosing products with lower sodium content

Try also adding fresh or dried herbs and spices to food rather than reaching for the salt shaker. Researcher Carolyn Ross[65] gave white sauce to 39 research participants who were over 60. The study participants were asked to compare three different formulations of the sauce at five different salt concentrations. One of the formulations had no added herbs, the second had just herbs, and the third had both herbs and chipotle seasoning. Their results showed the formulation with both herbs and chipotle seasoning made it difficult for the seniors to determine the amount of salt being used while the formulation with exclusively herbs did not. This research suggests it may be particularly important to add more spices to food as you get older. Even if you've never liked spicy food, it may be now you will enjoy it, because your sense of taste may be less strong.

If you are used to adding a lot of salt to your food or eating salty snacks, this can seem too difficult. It's best to reduce your salt intake bit by bit, giving your taste buds chances to adapt. Also seek out non-salty snacks, but don't reach for the high sugar ones instead!

I recently had a good example of how taste buds can adjust. I've always loved crisps (called chips in the USA). That salty taste ... mmm. Earlier this year my partner bought some "naked" crisps. They had no salt. I was dubious but decided to try them. I was surprised at how much I liked them. The crunchy texture was still there. Since then, we've always bought the crisps without salt. Recently I was travelling and bought a packet of crisps with salt, as that is all that was available. They tasted terrible – it felt like I was eating neat salt! Just shows how your taste buds can and do adjust. We haven't evolved to eat this amount of salt, so in reducing your salt intake you are going back to what your salt intake should be. It makes sense that the body will adapt to that.

The World Health Organisation lists some of the misconceptions people often have about salt and its response:

- "On a hot and humid day when you sweat, you need more salt in the diet:" There is little salt lost through sweat so there is no need for extra salt even on a hot and humid day, although it is important to drink a lot of water.

- "Sea salt is not 'better' than manufactured salt simply because it is 'natural.'" Regardless of the source of salt, it is the sodium in salt that causes bad health outcomes.

- "Foods high in salt taste salty." Some foods that are high in salt don't taste very salty because sometimes they are mixed with other things like sugars that mask the taste. It is important to read food labels to find out sodium levels.

High salt intake has also been linked to some cancers, particularly stomach cancer. But it is difficult to confirm a clear link because a high intake of salt often means a high intake of processed foods, which are also linked to cancer.

High salt consumption has also been linked to obesity. Action on Salt[66] is based at Queen Mary University of London (UK). Their website explains:

"Whilst salt is not a direct cause of obesity, it is a major influencing factor through its effect on soft drink consumption: salt makes you thirsty and increases the amount of fluid you drink. "

High salt intakes have also been linked to asthma[67] , dermatitis[68], autoimmune diseases[69] and gastrointestinal bloating[70].

The heartandstroke.ca website[71] (Canada) says:

"Keep in mind that just because a food claims to be low in sodium doesn't mean it's healthy. These foods may still be high in fat, sugar and other undesirable ingredients"

The evidence is clear: eating less salt is beneficial whatever your age.

Sugar

Lots of people aren't aware of how much sugar they consume. This is particularly true if you don't add sugar to hot drinks. This can lull you into a false sense of virtue about your sugar consumption.

Harvard Health[72] says:

"In the American diet, the top sources are soft drinks, fruit drinks, flavored yogurts, cereals, cookies, cakes, candy, and most processed foods. But added sugar is also present in items that you may not think of as sweetened, like soups, bread, cured meats, and ketchup."

You may like the taste of sugar, and you may think you need a certain amount in your diet. Do you need sugar for energy? Some time ago I met a woman who said to me: "Everyone needs some sugar for energy." I pointed out to her that if this were really true the human race would have died out a long time ago, as sugar as a food is a relatively recent development.

Your body runs on glucose. It is the simple sugar that cells use for energy, but that doesn't mean you need to feed it regular sugar. Blood sugar, which gives you the energy to do things, is not necessarily made from sugar in food. Your body has a process known as catabolism in which food is broken down and turned into energy for your body.

But the advertisers have done a good job. In the UK we had a long-running advertisement for a Mars Bar (a chocolate bar) whose slogan was "A Mars A Day Helps You Work Rest and Play". But is sugar really good for us?

Some scientists[73] have looked at what happens to your body after eating lots of sugar. After feeding some people lots of sugar, the participants said they felt really tired one hour after eating their sweet treats. They were experiencing a "sugar crash" after a "sugar rush". Some people also experience feeling jittery, and anxious or develop a headache with the sugar crash.

The science says you may feel better immediately after eating something sugary, but subsequently, you will feel worse. Many people are aware of this at least instinctively, because when the sugar crash hits, they reach for more sugar to get back to the high. In the long run, sugar doesn't give you more energy. It just sets you off on an unpleasant roller coaster of highs and lows.

Seeing sugar as a solution rather than a problem doesn't help you in the long run, even if you feel better immediately after eating sugar. Of course, diabetics experiencing hypoglycaemia should have sugar at that time.

There are different types of sugar. People often think that some sugars are OK for them, but let's see what the evidence says.

The main one you should be concerned about in this context is sucrose. Sucrose is the common sugar made from sugar cane or sugar beets. Fructose is a type of sugar found in fruit. Fructose has a much lower glycaemic index than sucrose. In practical terms this means that it has a less dramatic effect on blood sugar than sucrose does.

High fructose corn syrup is a highly processed sugar from corn. It is found in many processed foods and drinks, particularly in the USA. There have been a lot of health concerns[74] about it, so this is definitely not a good alternative to sugar.

Some people justify their sugar intake by using brown sugar, which has some minerals in it. But the quantities of minerals do not counteract the harm from the sugar, so it is not a healthy alternative.

Should you avoid all sucrose? In an ideal world, the answer to this is 'yes', but a small amount of sugar is OK for most people. There are some medical exceptions to this. But don't try to convince yourself that sugar gives you energy or is necessary for your survival. It definitely is not. Reducing your sugar consumption will undoubtedly help your health and well-being.

Sucrose is usually regarded as empty calories. It contains no nutrients that the body needs. It absolutely contributes to weight problems. Consuming sugar can mean that you eat less nutrient-dense food, because you have filled up with sugary food.

Robert Lustig[75] of the University of California (USA) sums up some of the dangers when he writes:

"Too much sugar causes diabetes, heart disease, fatty liver disease and tooth decay. When consumed in excess, it's a toxin. And it's addictive – just like alcohol."

It's definitely not a good idea to try to quickly reduce your sugar intake. But also, don't kid yourself that you are reducing your sugar intake when you're not.

Artificial sweeteners

If you don't want to give up sugar, you may think you are doing the right thing by replacing it with artificial sweeteners, particularly if you are trying to lose weight.

Yet the research does not support this. Dr Michael Greger of nutritionfacts.org[76] explains:

"... population studies tying consumption of artificial sweeteners, mainly in diet sodas, with increased risk of developing obesity, metabolic syndrome, and type 2 diabetes. But an association is not causation. You've got to put it to the test. If you give obese individuals the amount of sucralose found in like a can of diet soda, they get a significantly higher blood sugar spike in response to a sugar challenge, requiring significantly more insulin – 20% higher insulin levels in the blood – suggesting sucralose causes insulin resistance, potentially helping to explain the links between artificial sweetener consumption and the development of diabetes, heart disease, and stroke."

Do artificial sweeteners actually help you lose weight? Most artificial sweeteners have zero or few calories, but this doesn't mean they will help you lose weight.

Researchers[77] from the University of Manitoba (Canada) published a study in the Canadian Medical Association Journal. They conducted a systematic review of 37 studies that followed over 400,000 people for an average of 10 years. Only seven of these studies were randomized controlled trials (the gold standard in clinical research), involving 1003 people followed for 6 months on average.

The trials did not show a consistent effect of artificial sweeteners on weight loss. In fact, almost the opposite. The longer observational studies showed a link between the consumption of artificial sweeteners and relatively higher risks of weight gain and obesity, high blood pressure, diabetes, heart disease and other health issues.

Professor Ruopeng An[78] of the University of Illinois (USA) examined the dietary habits of more than 22,000 U.S. adults. He found that diet-beverage consumers may compensate for the absence of calories in their drinks by eating extra food that is loaded with sugar, sodium, fat and cholesterol.

An said:

"It may be that people who consume diet beverages feel justified in eating more, so they reach for a muffin or a bag of chips ... Or perhaps, in order to feel satisfied, they feel compelled to eat more of these high-calorie foods."

James Brown[79] of Aston University (UK) says:

"Based on current evidence, it's generally agreed that using artificial sweeteners is associated with increased body weight – though researchers aren't quite certain whether sweeteners directly cause this to happen."

Researchers[80] from the University of Manitoba (Canada) said:

"We found that data from clinical trials do not clearly support the intended benefits of artificial sweeteners for weight management."

The research is very conclusive. Don't use artificial sweeteners to help you lose weight.

Associate Professor James Brown[81] of Aston University (UK) says:

"Sweeteners have long been suggested to be bad for our health. Studies have linked consuming too many sweeteners with conditions such as obesity, type 2 diabetes and cardiovascular disease."

He goes on to say that there is a slight increase in cancers in people who consume the most compared with those who consume the least

Another study[82] put it much more strongly than this. Researchers analysed data from 102,865 French adults participating in the NutriNet-Santé study. The researchers found that enrollees consuming larger quantities of artificial sweeteners, particularly aspartame and acesulfame-K, had a higher risk of overall cancer than non-consumers. The researchers say:

"Our findings do not support the use of artificial sweeteners as safe alternatives for sugar in foods or beverages"

So, there you have it. It's best not to use artificial sweeteners or buy foods that contain them.

Water

Not drinking enough fluids can have all sorts of effects on the body. Some older people reduce fluid intake, so they don't need to go for a pee so often but doing that has all sorts of health implications. If you allow yourself to become even mildly dehydrated, you are likely:

- To have higher blood pressure.[83]

- To have harder and smaller stools that are difficult to pass. You may become constipated.

- To become tired, dizzy and confused.

- Your skin may become itchy and uncomfortable.

Your brain on unhealthy food

There is more and more evidence that the more badly you eat, the more you are driven to eat badly. Your brain is literally changed.

Researchers[84] at the Max Planck Institute for Metabolism Research in Cologne (Germany), in collaboration with Yale University (USA), have now shown that foods with a high fat and sugar content change your brain: If you regularly eat even small amounts of them, the brain learns to consume precisely these foods in the future.

Twice a day the researchers gave one group of volunteers a small yoghurt that was high in fat and sugar. The other group received yoghurts that contained the same number of calories but were low in fat and sugar. The volunteer's brain activity was measured before and during the eight weeks.

The brain's response to high-fat and high-sugar foods was greatly increased in the group that ate the high-sugar and high-fat pudding after eight weeks. This particularly activated the dopaminergic system, the region in the brain responsible for motivation and reward. The brain rewired itself through the consumption of these yoghurts. People talk about being addicted to fast food or to some individual product. This research suggests that framing it like this may be close to the truth.

The researchers didn't test what would happen to the participants' brains if they stopped eating those yoghurts. It seems likely that over time the brain would rewire itself again.

If this is true, it means that when you first change your diet away from one that is high in fat and sugar, your brain will prompt you to want those unhealthy foods. If you persist in eating healthily, it is likely that the brain prompts will weaken. You need to take a long view. When it is difficult initially, recognise that eventually it will become a lot easier. If you've ever given up tobacco or alcohol or some addictive drug, you will recognise this process.

If you are struggling in the early days, don't just think you can't face this for the rest of your life. Remember this demand from your brain won't be this strong for the rest of your life.

When I talk to friends who generally eat well, they all say the same thing. If they start adding more processed food or sweet or salty food to their diet regularly, it becomes harder to resist. They start to look for it and feel deprived if they don't have it. When they cut these things out, the body (or perhaps I should say mind) adapts to this again and these foods become less tempting.

Putting it all together

There are lots of suggestions and recommendations in this chapter. I don't recommend trying to implement them all in one go. Instead, start with the one or ones that you know you will find easiest to implement.

You may look at all this and think it's going to be boring and tasteless. That's not true. This sort of food can be extremely tasty. Also remember that eating in this way will almost certainly decrease your desire for high-fat and high-sugar foods. They'll become less appealing and less satisfying to eat. Eating this way will also make you happier. I'll talk more about this in the chapter on happiness.

You may be surprised I haven't talked about calories, particularly given how many people are overweight or obese. But if you focus on increasing the amount of fruit, veggies and beans in your diet, you will automatically decrease the calories you consume.

I haven't mentioned fibre either. Again, this is because if you eat more veggies, beans and fruit you will automatically eat more fibre.

If you want to improve your diet, change slowly. Focus On Nutrition (Harvard Medical School) says:

"By the time you are 40, you'll have eaten some 40,000 meals—and lots of snacks besides. Give yourself time to change, targeting one item a week... Take a long-range view. Don't get down on yourself if you slip up or "cheat" from time to time. Don't worry about every meal, much less every mouthful. Your nutritional peaks and valleys will balance out if your overall dietary pattern is sound."

Constipation

Many older people struggle with constipation. Constipation can make you feel sluggish and headachy. It can also mean that going to the toilet is painful and distressing.

Causes of constipation

There are various reasons for constipation, so let's look at them.

Firstly, a poor diet. This means a diet that doesn't include fibre. You may think of fibre as meaning you have to eat wholemeal bread and brown rice and wholemeal pasta. These are important sources of fibre, but so are oats, fruit, vegetables and pulses (legumes). Be sure to add more fibre to your diet a little at a time so your body gets used to the change. Fibre is important, because it gives your stools bulk, making them easier to pass.

If you have irritable bowel disease or other similar problems, it may not be appropriate to increase your fibre intake. In this case, do talk to your medical practitioner about this.

Lack of adequate fluids can lead to stools that are difficult to pass. Lack of exercise can also lead to constipation. Yet another reason to move around as much as you can.

Some drugs may lead to constipation, such as antidepressants, antacids containing aluminium or calcium, antihistamines, diuretics, and anti-Parkinsonism drugs.

Certain medical conditions (such as hypothyroidism and diabetes) may also cause constipation, so it is worth consulting your medical practitioner if you start to experience constipation.

Laxatives

If you're taking laxatives regularly, you may want to think again. Regular laxative use may change the microbiome of the gut. This may affect nerve signalling from the gut to the brain or increase the production of intestinal toxins that may affect the brain.

A study[85] looked at 500,000 people in the UK with an average age of 57. None of them had a dementia diagnosis at the beginning of the study. 3.6% reported using over-the-counter laxatives most days of the week during the month before the study began. The participants were followed for around 10 years.

The study found that people who regularly used laxatives had a 51% increased risk of overall dementia compared to people who did not regularly use laxatives.

Researchers said:

"If our findings are confirmed, medical professionals could encourage people to treat constipation by making lifestyle changes such as drinking more water, increasing dietary fiber and adding more activity into their daily lives."

As we know from other research, making these lifestyle changes won't only alleviate constipation and reduce your chance of getting dementia, they also have many other important health benefits.

Putting on weight as you get older

In an earlier chapter, I quoted from the United Nations website[86] that four lifestyle changes could result in an 80% reduction in the chronic diseases associated with old age. Maintaining a healthy weight is one of these.

Adults in the UK[87] are now putting on 0.5kg to 1.0kg (1.1 lb to 2.2 lb) of weight every year. This may not sound much but that gradually adds up to more and more excess weight. And remember this is what happens to most people. You could be putting on more than that. Carrying unnecessary weight has health and well-being implications. It's not just about how you look.

Why do I put on weight as I get older?

As people get older, they often put on weight. They assume this is a normal, natural state of affairs. They know that their metabolism slows as they get older. They know that's why they are putting on weight. But is it really true?

Your metabolism does slow with age, but not by the huge amount that you may think. Researchers[88] from Pennington Biomedical Research Center (USA) studied how metabolism changes with age. They analysed the average calories burned by more than 6,600 people as they went about their daily lives. The participants' ages ranged from one week old to 95 years, and they lived in 29 different countries.

They found that metabolisms doesn't start to decline again until after age 60. Even then, the slowdown is gradual, only 0.7 percent a year. Much, much less than most people think.

So yes, your metabolism does slow down, but it's a small amount each year and is no excuse for piling on the pounds. You do need to take this into account in what you eat and stay as active as possible.

As you get older, are you tending to exercise less? This often happens because people believe this is what they should do as they get older. They think it's time to take it easy, rest more and do less. There is a grain of truth in this. Your ability to recover from vigorous exercise gets less as you get older, so you may need to take more time between sessions or run shorter distances. But the amount you need to ease back is often wildly exaggerated.

You will consume additional calories with exercise, but more importantly, you will retain muscle mass. There are lots of benefits to this – you will find all sorts of everyday tasks easier and be less likely to fall or develop dementia. One important benefit is that it takes more calories for your body to maintain muscle than it does to maintain fat. So, if you have an extra 10 lb of muscle, you will need more calories than if you have an extra 10 lb of fat, even when you are just sitting around.

If you spend a lot of time watching television, you need to consume fewer calories. If you are passionate about sedentary hobbies, you need to eat less. Playing bridge, doing intricate embroidery, knitting for charity or tracing your family history may stimulate your brain and fill your days with passion and pleasure, but these activities don't use that much physical energy. So, you need to eat less if you don't want to gain weight. Better still, take up some extra activities that are more vigorous.

Can eating become a habit?

As people get older, they often eat more and more from habit – they know what they like and what suits them. They may eat according to the clock. When asked; "Are you hungry?", they may immediately look at a watch or clock to decide the answer.

Because it's 11 am, do you decide that you'll have a milky coffee and a couple of biscuits (cookies)? That's just what happens at 11 am. Do you always have a pudding or other dessert with your dinner? Do you always have bread with soup? Do you always have a bar of chocolate or a couple of glasses of wine in the evening? Perhaps we shouldn't call it a decision, as it's so automatic. So, when someone asks: "Are you hungry?", don't look at your watch, but check out how you feel.

When you notice it's your normal lunchtime, stop and think about what you want to eat according to how hungry you are. This will take practice and perseverance.

Try committing yourself to cooking one new healthy meal a week. If you mainly buy s ready-cooked meals, commit to choosing something new each week. If you regularly eat out, try something different from the menu at least once a month. Not everything will be a success, but this way you keep your culinary horizons expanded. That helps to keep your mental horizons expanded too. These actions will start to break up those automatic eating habits.

People who are at home all the time will often eat from boredom. The food is there, and they are a little bored, so a handful of this or a couple of that helps break up the boredom. If you eat from boredom, you need to find other things to do to fill up your life.

A study[89] of patients attending a UK hospital-based obesity service shows no difference in weight loss between those under 60 years old and those from 60 to 78 years old.

Lead author Dr Thomas Barber said:

"Weight loss is important at any age, but as we get older we're more likely to develop the weight-related co-morbidities of obesity. Many of these are similar to the effects of aging, so you could argue that the relevance of weight loss becomes heightened as we get older, and this is something that we should embrace."

All of this is sound advice. But remember that the big change is the mental shift: understanding that you don't have to get fatter as you get older. You know that your metabolism slows a bit, but that doesn't mean you have to put on a lot of weight.

Weight gain as you get older is not just about vanity either. Weighing more has a detrimental effect on your health and well-being.

Waist circumference

As well as your weight, you need to keep an eye on your waist circumference. The UK charity the British Heart Foundation[90] says:

"Waist circumference is a good measure of fat around your middle. This type of fat builds up around your organs, and is linked to high blood fat levels, high blood pressure and diabetes. A larger waist usually also means there is excess fat inside your organs. When this happens in your liver, for example, it pumps out too much fat and sugar into the blood, increasing your risk of coronary heart disease and diabetes."

Is your waist circumference a cause for concern? Here is what the research says:

Men, low risk: below 94cm (37in)

Men, high risk: 94–102cm (37-40in)

Men, very high risk: more than 102cm (40in)

Women, low risk: below 80cm (31.5in)

Women, high risk: 80–88cm (31.5-34.6in)

Women, very high risk: more than 88cm (34.6in)

These figures[91] are for "people of white European, black African, Middle Eastern and mixed origin.

"For men of African Caribbean, South Asian, Chinese and Japanese origin, a waist circumference below 90cm (35.4in) is low risk, and more than that is 'very high risk' (there isn't a 'high risk' category). For women from these groups, below 80cm (31.5in) is low risk, and anything above is very high risk."

So, get that tape measure out and check what your waist circumference is.

Tips to help you lose weight

Research shows that for many people dieting doesn't work. You may lose weight, but you are very likely to put the weight back on eventually. Dieting demands willpower. It's hard to have willpower all the time. But without an alternative many people keep returning to dieting and hoping for a different outcome.

I've written a book "190 Weight Loss Hacks: How to lose weight naturally and permanently without stress"[92]. It will give you lots of simple strategies you can use to lose weight without dieting. The vast majority of these are backed by scientific research about what really works. There are bound to be two or three strategies that will work for you.

Alcohol

Alcohol is often considered to be a problem for young, irresponsible people, but there is mounting evidence that many older people experience problems around alcohol.

Tony Rao[93], Visiting Lecturer in Old Age Psychiatry, King's College London (UK) says:

"Ageing is difficult. Older people are more likely to have chronic pain and have difficulty with mobility. And they are also more likely to experience bereavement and social isolation. Some people turn to alcohol for help, but this merely introduces a range of additional problems."

According to the 2023 Canada's Guidance on Alcohol and Health[94], 3–6 standard drinks a week represent a moderate risk to your health. After that, the more you drink, the more you increase your risk of seven types of cancer, most types of cardiovascular diseases, liver disease and violence. The bottom line is that, when it comes to alcohol and your health, less is better.

As you age, alcohol consumption can make existing health problems worse and have dangerous interactions with some medications. Alcohol tends to have more effect on the body as you age too, so most people should actually be drinking less.

The UK Mental Health Foundation[95] says:

"Too much alcohol can lead to low mood and anxiety. It can also cause sleep problems, dizziness, and memory problems and damage your liver, heart and brain over time. As we age, our bodies become more sensitive to alcohol, so it's likely to affect you more than younger people."

The US National Institute on Aging[96] says that drinking too much alcohol over a long time can:

- "Lead to some kinds of cancer, liver damage, immune system disorders, and brain damage.

- "Worsen some health conditions such as osteoporosis, diabetes, high blood pressure, stroke, ulcers, memory loss, and mood disorders.

- "Make some medical conditions hard for doctors to accurately diagnose and treat. For example, alcohol causes changes in the heart and blood vessels. These changes can dull pain that might be a warning sign of a heart attack.

- "Cause some older people to be forgetful and confused — symptoms that could be mistaken for signs of Alzheimer's disease or a related dementia."

A study by researchers from Anglia Ruskin University[97] (UK) followed 333,259 people who drank alcohol for around 7 years. The study analysed all incidents where participants had been hospitalised because of cardiovascular events.

Lead author Dr Rudolph Schutte said:

"Among drinkers of beer, cider and spirits in particular, even those consuming under 14 units a week had an increased risk of ending up in hospital through a cardiovascular event involving the heart or the blood vessels. While we hear much about wine drinkers having lower risk of coronary artery disease, our data shows their risk of other cardiovascular events is not reduced. Biases embedded in epidemiological evidence mask or underestimate the hazards associated with alcohol consumption."

Alcohol and medication

The US National Institute on Aging[98] cautions:

- "If you take aspirin and drink, your risk of stomach or intestinal bleeding increases.

- "When combined with alcohol, cold and allergy medicines (antihistamines) may make you feel very sleepy.

- "Alcohol used with large doses of acetaminophen, a common painkiller, may cause liver damage.

- "Some medicines, such as cough syrups and laxatives, have a high alcohol content. If you simultaneously drink alcohol, that will add to the effects.

- "Alcohol used with some sleeping pills, pain pills, or anxiety/anti-depression medicine can be deadly."

But what about red wine?

Many people justify the amount they drink on the basis that research shows some alcohol (particularly red wine) is beneficial. When researchers first proposed this, the idea spread like wildfire. This is not surprising, as it gave people a justification for what they were doing.

William Porter[99], author of the book Alcohol Explained, says:

"Alcohol is a poisonous chemical. It kills living things (which is why it is used in hand sanitiser) ... Fruits are a natural part of the human diet and contain vitamins and minerals in abundance that keep us feeling well and healthy. So of course red wine, being primarily made up of grape juice, contains many things that are good for us. So it is easy to say that this, that or the other in red wine is good for us. But that is the grape side and not the alcohol side of it."

He then goes on to argue:

"The moderate drinkers [in the scientific studies] tend to be wealthier, more educated, smoke less, live in nicer areas, are less likely to have been in prison, less likely to be overweight, and in general, are better off than both people who drink a lot and those who say that they never drink. "

He sees this lifestyle, not the moderate drinking as responsible for the health discrepancies. In other words, you could get all the benefits by drinking non-alcoholic grape juice without the downside of alcohol consumption.

Even if you don't agree with his analysis and want to believe that red wine is beneficial, do remember that the researchers are talking about moderate drinking. The US Centers for Disease Control[100] defines this as:

"1 drink or less on a day for women or 2 drinks or less on a day for men."

This is not a lot. Many people find it difficult to stop at this level of drinking, so it may be better off not routinely drinking alcohol at all.

If you drink alcohol regularly, you need to have days when you don't drink any. It's not enough just to believe that you could do that if you wanted to! You need to monitor how much you drink. If you are drinking alcohol regularly at home, it is easy for portion size to grow, so that you are drinking far more than the 1 or 2 glasses a day suggests.

Smoking

In an earlier chapter, I quoted from the United Nations website[101] that four lifestyle changes could result in an 80% reduction in the chronic diseases associated with old age. Quitting smoking is one of these important four changes.

The US Centers for Disease Control[102] is in no doubt:

"Quitting smoking is one of the most important actions people can take to improve their health. This is true regardless of their age or how long they have been smoking."

They go on to say:

"Quitting smoking .... benefits people already diagnosed with coronary heart disease or COPD ... Quitting smoking is the single best way to protect family members, coworkers, friends, and others from the health risks associated with breathing secondhand smoke."

Smoking and cancer

Everyone is aware that smoking causes lung cancer, but did you know that it's also implicated in many other cancers? The US government CDC[103] says:

"Cigarette smoking can cause cancer almost anywhere in the body. Cigarette smoking causes cancer of the mouth and throat, esophagus, stomach, colon, rectum, liver, pancreas, voicebox (larynx), trachea, bronchus, kidney and renal pelvis, urinary bladder, and cervix, and causes acute myeloid leukemia."

Researchers from Wake Forest School of Medicine[104] (USA) found that nicotine creates an environment in the lungs that is ripe for metastatic growth. Metastatic growth is when the cancer spreads from its original site to other sites in the body. If you smoke, the cancer finds this an easier process. The researchers found that cigarette smoking is associated with a higher incidence of breast cancer spread, or metastasis, lowering the survival rate by 33% at diagnosis.

Smoking and diabetes

The risk of developing type 2 diabetes[105] is 30% to 40% higher for people who currently smoke than for those who don't.

Smoking and weight

Many people are reluctant to give up smoking because they are afraid that they will put on a lot of weight. Smoking lowers your appetite. Having something in your mouth may be soothing, so eating can become a substitute for smoking. Eating may become your way of dealing with negative emotions.

The smokefree.gov[106] website (USA) says:

"If you are worried about gaining weight after you quit, try to remember:

"Quitting smoking is the best thing you can do for your health right now ... You can do things to help prevent weight gain while you become smokefree. If you do gain weight after quitting, it doesn't have to be forever. There are healthy ways you can lose the weight."

Smoking and mental health

The influential US Centers for Disease Control[107] says:

"Quitting smoking cigarettes is associated with lower levels of anxiety, depression, and stress, as well as improved positive mood and quality of life."

This may seem surprising, but this is the conclusion after their scientist have looked at all the research in this area. Initially, it will probably lead you to feel more stressed, but hold on to the thought that eventually your mental health will be better.

What happens when you give up smoking?

Many people who smoke want to give up. Here's information on what happens to your body after you smoke that last cigarette. This information shows how quickly you can benefit from giving up smoking. Stop smoking now and see the changes that can happen in your health over the next year, the next five years and so on.

According to the American Heart Association[108] and the U.S. Surgeon General, this is how your body starts to recover when you quit smoking:

In the first 20 minutes: your blood pressure and heart rate recover from the nicotine-induced spikes.

After 12 hours: the carbon monoxide levels in your blood return to normal.

After 2 weeks: your circulation and lung function begin to improve.

After 1 to 9 months: clear and deeper breathing gradually returns; you have less coughing and shortness of breath; you regain the ability to cough productively instead of hacking. This cleans your lungs and reduces your risk of infection.

After 1 year: your risk of coronary heart disease is reduced by 50 percent.

After 5 years: Your risk of cancer of the mouth, throat, esophagus, and bladder are cut in half. Your risk of cervical cancer and stroke return to normal.

After 10 years: You are half as likely to die from lung cancer. Your risk of larynx or pancreatic cancer decreases.

After 15 years: your risk of coronary heart disease is the same as a non-smoker's.

What about e-cigarettes?

If you read this and decide to stop smoking, don't change to e-cigarettes, as these aren't necessarily any less harmful. E-cigarettes do not produce tar or carbon monoxide, two of the most harmful elements in tobacco smoke, so you may think that changing to them is a step in the right direction.

They can be used as a stage on the way to stopping altogether. The UK NHS[109] says:

" ... using a vaping product as part of a quit attempt in local stop smoking services had some of the highest quit success rates"

But note that vaping products are used as part of an overall strategy and not on their own. Sadly, some people take up vaping with no real intention of quitting. They may feel it is harmless, but is it really?

A Vaping Q&A[110] from Johns Hopkins Bloomberg School of Public Health (USA) is categorical:

"No one should be vaping unless they are a cigarette user trying to quit using cigarettes."

Researchers[111] at the same university found that vaping aerosols contain thousands of unknown chemicals and substances not disclosed by manufacturers, including industrial chemicals and caffeine.

E-cigarettes are usually flavoured, and this may be detrimental too, although much of the research on flavours has been done on the basis of people eating them.

How to stop smoking

I used to smoke over 40 cigarettes a day and tried several times before finally succeeding. A few years later a friend who smoked was staying for Christmas. I decided to have "just one". I was curious what it would be like assuming I would hate it. But it didn't happen like that – I absolutely loved it. I made her promise me she wouldn't give me another one no matter how much I begged her. This incident made it very clear to me that I had to be an ex-smoker or someone who smoked 40+ a day. Fortunately, I chose the ex-smoker route.

High-quality evidence[112] from over 300 studies of over 250,000 people shows that receiving stop-smoking counselling increases long-term quit rates.

Many governments, health charities and health agencies offer free support for those who want to stop smoking. In the USA the smokefree.gov[113] website offers text support. They have different programmes depending on where you are with your journey to stop smoking. For example, the Daily Challenges program might send you a text suggesting you delay your first cigarette by one hour. This helps you gradually to cut down. The Smokefree program for people ready to stop smoking completely might send you this text: "Cravings can be triggered by seeing other people smoking. Spend time in places where smoking isn't allowed. Try malls, museums, or the movies."

The part of the website[114] aimed at people who are 60+ is well worth exploring if you are over 60. They also have a website section[115] where you build your own plan for stopping smoking.

The UK NHS also offers stop-smoking services, including one-to-one and group stop-smoking sessions. Jennifer Percival, who trains stop-smoking advisers, says that using treatments together

"Overall, you're up to 3 times more likely to stop smoking for good if you use a combination of stop smoking treatment and receive support from an NHS Stop Smoking Service."

If you're in another country, check out what your government or other agencies offer you.

A smartphone smoke-free app might be helpful. Some are paid for, but reputable charities and government agencies offer free ones in many countries. Some of these apps offer help tailored specifically for you. These are based on your smoking patterns, moods, motivation to quit, and quitting goals. You can tag the locations and times of day when you need extra support. Search the app store using the phrase "smoke-free app".

Giving up smoking can be one of the very best things you can do for your health, for your finances and for those who regularly share your space. Remember the evidence is clear. You should probably get support rather than trying to do it on your own.

Exercise

In an earlier chapter, I quoted from the United Nations website[116] that four lifestyle changes could result in an 80% reduction in the chronic diseases associated with old age. Exercise is one of these.

Exercise should be an important part of your plan to age well. Professor Stuart Phillips[117] of McMaster University, Canada says:

"Greater levels of physical activity are associated with so many health benefits it is hard to comprehend. From mental health to cancer risk, everything gets better the more physically active you are. I cannot think of a single solitary health behavior that, if adhered to, does as much for your health as being physically active. Move so you don't lose as you age!"

The American Heart Association[118] says:

"It's true, 70 is the new 60... but only if you're healthy. People who are physically active and at a healthy weight live about seven years longer than those who are not active and are obese. And the important part is that those extra years are generally healthier years! Staying active helps delay or prevent chronic illnesses and diseases associated with aging. So active adults maintain their quality of life and independence longer as they age."

The UK NHS[119] enthusiastically says:

"Exercise is the miracle cure we've always had, but for too long we've neglected to take our recommended dose. Our health is now suffering as a consequence. This is no snake oil. Whatever your age, there's strong scientific evidence that being physically active can help you lead a healthier and happier life.

"People who exercise regularly have a lower risk of developing many long-term (chronic) conditions, such as heart disease, type 2 diabetes, stroke, and some cancers.

"Research shows that physical activity can also boost self-esteem, mood, sleep quality and energy, as well as reducing your risk of stress, clinical depression, dementia and Alzheimer's disease."

Exercise even affects your gut biome. The complex mix of bacteria that live in your gut affects not only your digestion but also your ability to fight infection. It's also been shown to affect your mood. A healthy gut biome with a wide range of different types of bacteria is vitally important for your well-being.

A study from the University of Calgary (Canada)[120] of middle-aged adults found that physical activity of moderate duration (greater than 150 minutes per week) increased both the richness and diversity of the gut microbiomes compared to study participants who exercised less. The study found that how hard you exercised during that 150-plus minutes didn't have any additional benefits for the gut biome. Of course, it may be beneficial for other reasons.

I could go on and on, quoting authorities and studies about the benefits of exercise to help prevent the chronic diseases of ageing, to help you live a longer and happier life. But I hope I've already convinced you that whatever else you do in your life, you need to take exercise. You probably need to take more exercise than you are doing now. But this idea may make you very nervous.

Is it safe to exercise as I get older?

If you're new to exercise, you may wonder if you should be doing any at all. The advice from experts is very clear. Chhanda Dutta[121] of the US National Institute on Aging says:

"Exercise is almost always good for people of any age"

The US National Institute on Aging[122] is categorical that even if you have a health condition like heart disease, arthritis, chronic pain, high blood pressure, or diabetes, you can still exercise. They also say that exercise may in fact help these conditions.

Assistant Professor of Geriatrics and Gerontology Alicia I. Arbaje[123] puts it very clearly:

"A lot of the symptoms that we associate with old age - such as weakness and loss of balance - are actually symptoms of inactivity, not age."

The World Health Organization[124] (WHO) agrees. Their advice on physical activity for adults aged 65 years and above:

" Same as for adults [under 65]; and as part of their weekly physical activity, older adults should do varied multicomponent physical activity that emphasizes functional balance and strength training at moderate or greater intensity, on 3 or more days a week, to enhance functional capacity and to prevent falls."

Helen Branthwaite of Staffordshire University (UK) has written a really interesting article[125] entitled "Four ways older adults can get back to exercising – without the worry of an injury ". In it, she writes:

"Maintaining muscle is important for many reasons. As we age, frailty can make it more difficult for us to be independent and do the things we need to do each day – from going shopping to meeting our friends. Being active maintains a healthy musculoskeletal system whilst also protecting us from some diseases, such as type 2 diabetes. Research also shows that strong active muscles can help prevent falls and lower injury risk."

If you have back pain, you may think that exercise is not suitable for you. Research now suggests you should exercise if you can. A systematic review[126] of the literature concluded that an exercise programme that combines muscular strength, flexibility and aerobic fitness is beneficial for people with chronic low back pain. Of course, if your back pain is caused by a tumour, an inflammatory disorder, a deformity and so on, it may not be suitable. But for the vast majority of people, it is. Strength training will increase the strength of the muscles that support your back and give you a greater range of movement. Aerobic exercise increases the blood flow and nutrients to the soft tissues in the back, improving the healing process and reducing stiffness.

The American Heart Association[127] says:

"Even if you've been sedentary for years, today is the day you can begin to make healthy changes in your life. Set a reachable goal for today. You can work up toward the recommended amount by increasing your time as you get stronger. Don't let all-or-nothing thinking keep you from doing what you can every day."

How much exercise should I do?

The US government Centers for Disease Control says that adults aged 65 and over need:

- At least 150 minutes a week (for example, 30 minutes a day, 5 days a week) of moderate-intensity activity such as brisk walking. Or they need 75 minutes a week of vigorous-intensity activity such as hiking, jogging, or running.

- At least 2 days a week of activities that strengthen muscles.

- Activities to improve balance such as standing on one foot about 3 days a week.

The website also says:

"If chronic conditions affect your ability to meet these recommendations, be as physically active as your abilities and conditions allow."

Researchers from the University of Cambridge[128] (UK) found that one in ten early deaths could be prevented if everyone managed at least half the recommended level of physical activity. That's just 75 minutes a week. This would be sufficient to lower the risk of diseases such as heart disease, stroke and a number of cancers.

Fear of falling and improving your balance

Balance is vitally important, but it is something you probably took for granted when you were younger. As you get older, balance can get more problematic. If your balance is weak, you are more likely to stumble and fall.

Around half of older people are afraid of falling. Ironically, being afraid of falling may double your chances of actually falling[129]. In the UK around a third of people 65 and over fall at least once a year.

According to Public Health England[130] around 20% of patients with hip fractures end up in long-term residential care within a year of the fracture. In the USA, an older person dies from falling every 19 minutes[131]. Also, in the US[132] falls are the leading cause of fatal and nonfatal injuries among older adults, causing hip fractures, head trauma, and death.

These are shocking figures. A lot of falls happen because people have poor balance. If your only form of exercise is walking (and maybe a bit of gardening), you are more likely to fall. When older people fall, they often lose confidence and become less independent. If you are afraid of falling (and remember half of older people are), you are likely to limit in some ways what you do. You're likely to be nervous of going to new places. You may also be nervous about going to existing places, particularly if you feel people are pressing you to move faster. This can mean your world gets smaller and you get less confident.

Much of the advice about how to prevent falls involves making the environment safer.

The UK NHS[133], for example, offers this advice for avoiding falls at home:

- immediately mopping up spillages

- removing clutter, trailing wires and frayed carpet

- using non-slip mats and rugs

- making sure all rooms, passages and staircases are well-lit

- organising your home so that climbing, stretching and bending are kept to a minimum, and to avoid bumping into things

- getting help to do things you're unable to do safely on your own

- not walking on slippery floors in socks or tights

- not wearing loose-fitting, trailing clothes that might trip you up

- wearing well-fitting shoes that are in good condition and support the ankle

- taking care of your feet by trimming your toenails regularly and seeing a GP or chiropodist about any foot problems

Of course, these are important, but focusing on these misses one of the most important things people can do to reduce their chances of falling and to reduce their chances of injury if they do fall. The NHS goes on to say (much less prominently) that doing regular strength exercises and balance exercises can improve your strength and balance and reduce your risk of having a fall.

Balance problems can be caused by several different factors:

- Medications such as antidepressants, anticonvulsants, sedatives etc.

- Inner ear problems.

- Alcohol

- Medical conditions such as diabetes, heart disease, stroke, or problems with your vision, thyroid, nerves, or blood vessels can cause dizziness and other balance problems

These problems should, of course, be excluded by consulting your medical practitioner.

One of the biggest reasons for balance problems is frailty and lack of strength through not moving enough. This can easily be righted, and you can do some of these exercises while watching TV or waiting for a kettle to boil. If you search online for "exercises to help balance", you will find lots of videos. Commonly recommended exercises include:

- Lifting one foot behind you and holding it for 10 seconds (while holding the back of a chair if necessary)

- Lifting one front in front of you and holding for 10 seconds (while holding the wall in front of you if necessary)

- Walking toe to heel, moving the heel of one foot to touch the toe of the other foot and so on)

- Moving sideways in a slow and controlled manner

- Stepping up and down on to a stair

Catching a ball can be a fun thing to do and help improve your balance too.

The Youtube channel[134] from physical therapists Bob and Brad has lots of suitable resources, as does the channel by Dr Alyssa Kuhn[135].

The UK NHS 24's Scottish Centre for Telehealth and Telecare[136] have developed a programme for fall prevention. It has three levels depending on how frail you are.

These exercises should be viewed as a starting point if you are somewhat frail and uncertain. Hopefully as your body gets stronger and more reliable, you will want to do more and get fitter and stronger.

What about walking?

You've probably heard that you should be walking 10,000 steps a day. It's often said that this is what you need to do to lower your risk of disease and death.

The 10,000-step idea originated from a marketing campaign rather than being driven by research into health outcomes. A Japanese company (Yamasa Corporation) built an advertising campaign for their new step-tracker. The pedometer's name — Manpo-Kei means 10,000-step meter in English. It gave them a catchy marketing campaign.

So, do you need to do 10,000 steps a day or is it OK to do fewer?

A large study, led by the University of Massachusetts[137] (USA), followed over 2,000 middle-aged adults from different ethnic backgrounds over a period of 11 years. The researchers found that those taking at least 7,000 steps a day had a 50 to 70% lower risk of dying during the study period compared with those taking fewer than 7,000 steps a day.

The effective step target might be even lower in older women[138]. A 2019 study of 16,741 women with a mean age of 72 years found those who averaged around 4,400 steps per day had significantly lower mortality rates when they were followed up more than four years later, compared with the least active women in the study.

Researchers from the University of Sydney[139] (Australia) monitored 78,500 adults with wearable trackers. They found lowered risk of dementia, heart disease, cancer and death are associated with achieving 10,000 steps a day.

If you hardly walk anywhere, the idea of doing 10,000 steps each day may be an appalling idea. But don't despair, you just need to get started. Remember research shows that you get benefit even if you don't do anywhere near 10,000 steps.

Just make a start. Set your sights on walking every day and adding more steps each day. Could you add an extra 100 steps each day until you can celebrate walking 1000 steps every day? If that's too much, aim to add 100 steps every few days or even once a week. The important thing is that you do this and make consistent progress from the level you started at.

You will be doing a lot more than many older people, and you'll really be benefitting your health and well-being. But walking is not the panacea many think it is. Walking will reduce your risk of many life-changing illnesses, but it is not sufficient on its own to achieve everything that exercise can do for you.

Walking is a great exercise for your leg muscles, but it doesn't cover all the ways your legs can move. It exercises your leg muscles repeatedly in the same way. If you are walking on a smooth surface, it won't give the stability muscles in your trunk a workout either. Nor will it do much for your upper body.

This, of course, doesn't mean that you shouldn't monitor how many steps you take each day. It's just that you should be aware that this isn't all the exercise your body needs. But if you're largely inactive now, this may well be the place to start. You can then add other types of exercise later.

Nordic walking (walking with poles) is beneficial in ways that conventional walking isn't. The American Association of Retired Persons[140] (AARP) says:

"Nordic walking has ... been shown to strengthen and tone the upper-body muscles and improve balance and stability. Because of the subtle spinal rotation involved in planting and then trailing your poles behind you, this kind of trekking builds core strength, too, which in turn improves posture."

The importance of aerobic exercise

Aerobic exercise[141] lowers your risk of heart and circulatory diseases. If you already have a heart or circulatory disease, regular aerobic exercise can also stop them getting worse.

And the benefits don't stop there. Aerobic exercise has been shown to lift your mood, boost the immune system, help some people with asthma and help with weight control.

The UK British Heart Foundation[142] says:

"It's recommended you do at least 150 minutes a week of moderate-intensity aerobic exercise. "Moderate intensity means you feel warm and comfortably breathless. If you are new to exercise, build up gradually to 150 minutes. Start by doing five to 10 minutes each day. Listen to how your body feels the next day before doing more."

Moderate-intensity aerobic exercise includes:

- brisk walking

- water aerobics

- dancing

- gardening

- tennis doubles

- biking at a moderate pace

The CDC[143] gives a simple way to establish if you're engaged in moderate intensity exercise or vigorous-intensity exercise.

"In general, if you're doing moderate-intensity activity, you can talk but not sing during the activity. In general, if you're doing vigorous-intensity activity, you will not be able to say more than a few words without pausing for a breath."

In other words, if you can talk and sing, your activity doesn't count as being part of the 150 minutes a week.

Next time you do what you consider to be moderate-intensity aerobic activity, check if you can still sing. If you can, it probably doesn't count towards the 150 minutes of moderate-intensity aerobic activity you need to do. It can, of course, be beneficial for other reasons.

The importance of strength training

Strength training, also known as resistance training or weight training, is a vitally important component of any healthy ageing programme. Sadly, many people think it's something for vain young people who are obsessed with how their bodies look. In fact, regular strength training benefits your overall health in many ways.

Professor Frank Meyer and colleagues[144] found that 20 to 30 minutes of strength training, 2 to 3 times per week, has positive effects on risk factors for heart disease, cancer, diabetes, and osteoporosis. So, you'll be less likely to suffer from the chronic diseases of old age if you do resistance training.

Strength training can also help to improve your posture. Poor posture makes you look older (and possibly fatter) than you really are. It also gives you strong bones and means you are less likely to fall.

I regularly ride my bike – I use it as my main form of transport. Recently there was a lot of rain and big puddles. I rode through a puddle not realising that the water was hiding a large hole. I came off my bike, landing with a loud thwack. I hit my shoulder and elbow. I picked myself up gingerly, wondering if I'd broken anything. Fortunately, I hadn't. I say "fortunately", but I don't think I was just lucky. I am convinced that I didn't break anything because I weight-train regularly. The minor-injuries doctor who examined me agreed with that. You may not ride a bike, but the importance of weight training for older people still applies. It helps keep your bones strong, so you are less likely to injure yourself if you fall.

What are the best strength training exercises?

The answer to this question depends on your existing level of fitness. If you are relatively fit and active and want to start strength training, you will be able to do exactly the same beginner routines as other people, but you may need to adjust your weights or the rests you take between sets.

For most exercises, you will do 8 to 15 repetitions (often known simply as reps). You will do 2 to 3 sets, resting for 30 to 90 seconds between each set. So, for example, when you start you might do an exercise for 10 repetitions, then rest for a minute, then repeat this sequence two more times.

I see older people in the gym and often the weights they are using are too light. If the weight isn't heavy enough, it won't challenge your body. If you don't challenge your body, you won't see any improvement. If you don't see any improvement, you'll probably decide "The gym doesn't work for me" or "It's so boring". Making the right amount of effort means you see the improvement in your body. That motivates you to keep going back to the gym or enjoying your online workout.

Dr Michelle Jongenelis from the University of Melbourne[145] (Australia) says that most older people aren't doing enough exercise. She then goes on to say:

"And when older people do exercise, it tends not to be at a high enough intensity level to reap all the potential benefits."

So how do you know what weights you should be using? How heavy is heavy? "Heavy weights" are heavy for you, so it varies from person to person. How do you determine what that should be? It's really simple:

- Prioritise form rather than weight. Good form means that you are doing the exercise correctly. You are using the correct muscles for that exercise. It means being aware of how your ankles, knees and pelvis are aligned. It involves being aware of what your back and shoulders are doing. It means not using momentum to swing the weights or leaning back inappropriately. This means you start with light enough weights to ensure that you can maintain that good form.

- Choose a weight where the last 2 or 3 repetitions in any set are hard. You couldn't easily do any more with proper form.

- Aim to make progress, so that you gradually increase the weights you lift. You can also make progress by shortening the breaks between sets or increasing the number of repetitions in each set.

You may prefer to work out at home rather than go to the gym. I love the HASfit website[146] for this. They have a whole section of beginner workouts that you can do in the comfort of your own home often just using your own body weight or water bottles. And they're free!

They have a section[147] specifically for seniors or those with limited mobility.

- 10 Minute Improve Balance Workout – Stability Exercises – Balance Exercises – Balancing Exercise – Stability Workouts

- 10 Minute Low Impact Aerobic Workout – Low Impact Cardio Exercises – Cardiovascular Exercise – Cardio Workouts

- 15 Minute Exercise for Seniors, Elderly, Older People, or Limited Mobility

- 15 Minute Senior Workout – Low Impact Workout – Senior Exercises – Exercise for Elderly

- 20 Minute Exercise for Seniors and Anyone with Limited Mobility

- 30 Minute Exercise for Seniors, Elderly, & Older People

- 30 Minute Exercise for Seniors and Anyone with Limited Mobility

Some of the exercises allow you to sit in a chair while working out.

- 20 Minute Standing & Seated Exercise for Seniors, Obese, & Limited Mobility Workout

- 25 Minute Chair Exercises Sitting Down Workout

- 30 Minute Standing & Seated Exercise for Seniors, Obese, Plus Size, & Limited Mobility Workout

- 30 Minute Senior Workout Routines – Standing & Seated Chair Exercise for Seniors, Elderly, Older People

There are also exercises to help with sciatica, neck pain and back pain:

- 15 Minute Neck Exercises for Neck Pain Relief

- 18 Minute Sciatica Exercises for Leg Pain Relief

- 30 Minute Exercises for Lower Back and Hip Pain Relief

They also have a lot of workouts for more advanced people. In fact, they have suitable workouts for everyone.

Pilates

Pilates is a type of mind-body exercise developed in the early 20th century by German physical trainer Joseph Pilates. It involves a series of exercises for core stability, strength, and flexibility. The exercises are done with attention to muscle control, posture, and breathing.

An analysis[148] of 30 studies showed 27 of the 30 studies reported advantages of Pilates for the elderly. The areas where more advantages were reported were in balance, although some showed benefits in total strength and ability to perform normal daily activities. Many participants in these studies also reported improved mood, sleep and quality of life.

Pilates can be a great option for anyone who is new to exercise or nervous of doing very much. Its gentle nature can be reassuring. Pilates classes can also be very sociable and supportive.

Tai Chi

Tai chi is a practice that involves a series of slow gentle movements and physical postures, a meditative state of mind, and controlled breathing. Tai chi originated as an ancient martial art in China. Over the years, it has become more focused on health promotion and rehabilitation.

The US National Center for Complementary and Integrative Health[149] says that Tai Chi may help to improve balance and prevent falls in older adults and people with Parkinson's disease There is also some research suggesting it may be helpful in reducing lower-back pain, fibromyalgia, and knee osteoarthritis. The Center also says it may be beneficial for people with mild cognitive impairment and for cancer-related symptoms.

Yoga

Researchers from the University of Edinburgh[150] (Scotland) reviewed 22 studies that had investigated the effects of yoga on physical and mental well-being in older adults. They concluded that people who practised yoga had "improved balance, flexibility, leg strength, depression, sleep quality, vitality and perceived mental and physical health – compared with no activity."

Yoga was particularly effective at improving lower body strength and flexibility, and reducing depression.

Yoga has been shown to improve sleep in studies[151] of older adults and people with cancer. People also find that yoga is a very sociable activity and that group participants feel like they are part of a caring community. This can help some people feel less lonely. Yoga can also help you lose weight[152] if you need to. This seems to be not so much because of the actual activity, but because it promotes a healthy lifestyle as well.

Other forms of exercise

Of course, there are many other types of exercise. For example, swimming (outdoors or in a pool), racket sports, line dancing, cycling (outdoors and spin classes) and running can all form a small or large part of your exercise routine.

The important thing here is "routine" and "consistency". Find ways to incorporate exercise into your life, so it becomes normal. Vary the type of exercise you do, including strength, aerobic exercise, and flexibility and balance. Strive to make progress – don't be satisfied with doing the same activity with the same amount of effort every time. Vary your exercise programme, challenge yourself and set yourself mini-targets. And, of course, remember to celebrate your success and the milestones on your way to better health – but preferably not with lots of cake or alcohol!

Sleep

In the USA[153] half of seniors have insomnia. In Canada[154] almost half of seniors reported having trouble falling asleep at least some of the time, and almost 30% reported difficulty staying awake during normal waking hours at least some of the time. The figures are probably similar for many other countries.

Benefits of sleep

There's lots of information available about the importance of sleep for good health and well-being, so I don't feel I need to provide a lot of evidence for this here. Here's just one example of the research showing how important sleep is for older people.

Researchers from University College London[155] (UK) found that:

" ... sleeping for five hours or less at the age of 50, 60, and 70 was linked to a 30% to 40% increased risk of multimorbidity when compared with those who slept for up to seven hours."

Multimorbidity means that the person has more than two diseases, such as heart disease, diabetes and respiratory disease. The researchers followed the participants for 25 years, so lack of sleep can reliably be seen as leading to bad health. It's not just that being ill interferes with sleep.

Insomnia medication

Prescription sleeping pills may help you fall asleep more easily or stay asleep longer — or both. Some medication can have side effects. The Mayo Clinic[156] lists the following:

- Dizziness or lightheadedness, which may lead to falls

- Headache

- Diarrhoea or nausea

- Prolonged drowsiness, more so with drugs that help you stay asleep

- Severe allergic reaction

- Sleep-related behaviors, such as driving or eating when not fully awake

- Changes in thinking and behavior, such as hallucinations, agitation, trouble remembering events, suicidal thoughts and bizarre behavior

- Daytime memory and performance problems

For these reasons, you should look for other ways to improve your sleep first.

Sleep and other medication

Some medications can interfere with sleep. The Express Scripts Pharmacy[157] says:

- Ingredients found in asthma inhaler medication or common cold and cough medications can cause anxiety, jitteriness, or restlessness that can interfere with sleep.

- Prescription steroids and stimulant medications — used mostly to treat ADHD or help with weight loss — can make you feel energized and stimulate wakefulness.

- Even though beta-blockers can lower your heart rate and make you sleepy, they also can lower your body's melatonin levels, which may cause nightmares that wake you up.

- Some medications can cause night-time leg cramps, such as ACE-inhibitors used for blood pressure control and heart failure, as well as cholesterol medications.

- Alpha-blockers, used to treat high blood pressure or prostate enlargement, can deprive you of the rest you need by interfering with deep REM sleep.

- Any over-the-counter medicines that include caffeine, like weight-loss supplements and some pain medications, along with smoking-cessation aids that contain nicotine, will also cause wakefulness.

Do not just stop taking medication because of what you have read here, but consult your doctor if you feel your medication may be a problem.

Set regular hours

The UK NHS[158] advises:

"First of all, keep regular sleeping hours. This programmes the brain and internal body clock to get used to a set routine."

There will be days when this is not possible, but there will be many days when you can do this. It may need some planning and involve other members of your household. You will be doing them a favour if it encourages them to set regular hours too.

Sleep and exercise

We know exercise has many benefits, including helping you maintain a healthy weight and lift your mood. It's also been found to help reduce insomnia. Regular aerobic exercise[159] has been shown to help people fall asleep quicker, wake up less during the night and feel more rested the following morning. This is true for many different types of aerobic exercise, such as cycling, running, and even brisk walking.

Studies[160] have found that people who do resistance exercise regularly (around three sessions per week) have better subjective sleep quality. Subjective sleep quality means how well you think you have slept, rather than your sleep being monitored by scientists. Even just thinking you have good quality sleep can affect how well you perform throughout the day.

Regular resistance training may also help people with insomnia to fall asleep quicker and increase their sleep efficiency. The evidence is not totally clear on this, but resistance training has many other benefits, particularly for older people. Do resistance training (strength training) knowing you will reap many benefits, including the possibility of sleeping better.

You may have read that you shouldn't exercise in the evening because it will disturb your sleep. Research shows that for some people it actually helps them get to sleep. Researchers[161] don't understand why, but it may be linked to core body temperature. You can try exercising at different times of the day and find what works best for you.

Many people exercise less as they age, so this may be part of the reason that older people tend to suffer more from insomnia than younger people.

Sleep and light

There has been some interesting research on the role of light on sleep quality. A study of 400,000 people[162] found that a lack of daytime light exposure was a risk factor for depressive symptoms, poor mood, and insomnia. Some older people spend a lot of time indoors. They don't have to go out to work. Maybe friends and relatives visit them rather than the other way round. If this is you, you need to plan to go outside when the day is bright. It doesn't mean you have to walk far, although that would be good for you for other reasons. If you have a garden, you could just go and sit in it for a while in the late morning or after lunch, for example.

A review of 45 studies[163] focused on people living in a community setting and concluded that brighter light delivered in the morning was associated with self-reported sleep improvements. Brighter evening light exposure was associated with worse self-reported sleep.

The Centers for Disease Control[164] says:

- If you have trouble falling asleep, dim the lights 2 hours before you want to go to sleep.

- If you get sleepy too early in the evening, go into a well-lit area to feel more awake.

Worries & Gratitude

Worries can keep you awake. Avoid looking at or paying bills and similar jobs just before you plan to go to bed.

The Royal College Of Psychiatrists[165] (UK) suggests:

"If something is troubling you and there is nothing you can do about it right away, try writing it down before going to bed and then tell yourself to deal with it tomorrow."

Also, do a simple gratitude process. Before you go to sleep think of three things that have happened (or not happened) in the day and take a moment to name each one and feel grateful for it.

Use essential oils

Essential oils are also known as aromatherapy oils. Try essential oils, which are widely regarded as having beneficial effects on sleep. There is also now some scientific evidence[166] to support this.

The Royal College Of Psychiatrists[167] (UK) says:

"Take some time to relax properly before going to bed. Some people find aromatherapy helpful."

Here are some essential oils you can try:

- Lavender helps slow heart rate and relax muscles.

- Sweet marjoram is calming and helps to slow the mind.

- Chamomile and Sandalwood help to reduce anxiety.

- Ylang Ylang has a soothing effect that alleviates stress.

- Peppermint oil aids sleep, probably by reducing stress.

You can use these oils in various ways. For example:

- Put a few drops of oil on a tissue and inhale the vapour

- Add to a carrier oil and then rub on your hands

- Add to water and spray in your room or on your pillow

Sleep and meditation

The UK charity The Sleep Charity[168] recommends meditation before sleep. You can devise your own or use one of the many free meditations available on the internet – just search for "sleep meditation". You can also use apps that include sleep meditations. I particularly like Headspace[169] for this. Sleep meditations include ones that help you get to sleep initially, as well as ones that help you to get back to sleep in the night. It may take you a while to find one that works for you, but fortunately, lots of options are available.

Dental health & gum disease

G um problems - gingivitis and periodontitis - affect at least 20% of people[170] worldwide.

Gingivitis is when the gums become inflamed and may bleed. Periodontitis is when the problems have spread to the soft tissue and bone responsible for keeping your teeth in place.

At one time it was thought that gum disease was a localised problem affecting just the mouth. The most serious problem was believed to be loss of teeth, caused by periodontitis. But recent research shows that your gum health can affect your general health in surprising ways.

Periodontal disease[171] is likely to cause 44% increase in the risk of cardiovascular disease in people over 65. Type 2 diabetics with severe periodontal disease have 3.2 times greater mortality risk compared with individuals with no or mild periodontitis.

All this tells you that you need to pay attention to your gum health for the sake of your general health, as well as relieving pain and soreness in your mouth.

Improving your gum health

There is definitely a genetic component in gum disease, but there are also lots of actions you can take to improve your gum health, such as eating less sugar, avoiding tobacco and alcohol and reducing stress.

You need to also make sure you are using the correct techniques to clean your teeth. Here are some quick pointers:

- Brush your teeth for around two minutes, at least twice a day.

- Close your mouth slightly when you brush your top teeth, as it is easier to get your brush to the gum line.

- Using interdental brushes and floss can be really helpful. Use these before brushing your teeth, as they allow the toothpaste to penetrate more easily when debris has been cleared out of the way. Do this at least once a day.

- Do not rinse out the toothpaste once you've finished brushing your teeth.

- Go to the dentist and hygienist regularly and follow their advice.

You can find much more detailed information on the internet, including videos showing you exactly what to do.

Dry mouth

Your mouth may produce a little less saliva as you get older, leaving your mouth slightly dry. It may be that you are not generally drinking enough water, so this is always worth trying.

Medical problems that occur in older adults are very common causes of dry mouth. MedlinePlus[172] says:

"Many medicines, such as some used to treat high blood pressure, high cholesterol, pain, and depression, can reduce the amount of saliva you produce. This is probably the most common cause of dry mouth in older adults.

"Side effects from cancer treatment can cause dry mouth.

"Health conditions such as diabetes, stroke, and Sjögren syndrome can affect your ability to produce saliva."

If you are experiencing a dry mouth, you need to pay particular attention to cleaning your teeth and gums, as saliva helps to keep your mouth clean and healthy.

Happiness & purpose

B eing happy is not always easy. It can seem like the world is heading for disaster. Maybe you are worrying about your own health or that of a spouse. If you have children and grandchildren, you may feel unhappy about their situation. Personal relationships may be difficult – with family, friends or neighbours. Money may be a problem. You may be worrying about a political situation or what's happening to the natural world.

But happiness is important, both for your mental and emotional well-being and also for your physical well-being. Being happy doesn't just make you feel better, it also improves your health. Scientists are not totally sure of the mechanisms involved in this.

But it's clear that if you are happy, you are likely to eat healthier food, be more active and sleep better. You are likely to be more proactive about your health if you are feeling happy and optimistic.

A review of 15 studies[173] involving nearly 230,000 people found that an optimistic mindset was linked to a lower risk of heart attack and stroke, as well as a lower risk of death.

So, the question is how to have more happiness in your life? Let's have a look at strategies suggested by research.

Changing your focus

It can be easy to focus on things that make us unhappy. Maybe you go over and over an argument you've had with someone. Do you constantly worry about the future and think of all the bad things that can happen? The negative thoughts go round and round, making you less and less happy.

Aristotle said, "We are what we repeatedly do." If we are constantly unhappy and thinking about things that make us unhappy, the unhappiness gets reinforced and continues.

In 2011, US psychologist Martin Seligman came up with what he called the Perma model of well-being. PERMA stands for:

- Positive Emotion

- Engagement

- Relationships

- Meaning

- Achievement

Psychologist Glenn Williams[174] explains that:

"... this model is a helpful tool for understanding the various ways in which we can trigger more positive ways of thinking. These run the gamut from experiencing a positive emotion to being fully absorbed in a challenging task, creating a more loving connection with someone, trying to make sense of a difficult situation, or even simply ticking off jobs on a to-do list."

These five strategies can work for you. Maybe not all of them. You may find one works better than the others. Experiment and see which strategy (or strategies) lifts you up when you're down.

Pretending to be happy

Pretending you're happy can make you happier. A researcher from the University of South Australia[175] explains:

"In our research we found that when you forcefully practice smiling, it stimulates the amygdala – the emotional centre of the brain – which releases neurotransmitters to encourage an emotionally positive state.

"For mental health, this has interesting implications. If we can trick the brain into perceiving stimuli as 'happy', then we can potentially use this mechanism to help boost mental health."

So, give it a try. Smile even though you may be feeling down.

Food and happiness

If you eat poorly, it seems self-evident that it can affect your physical health. Now research is showing that what you eat can also affect your mental health – your mood and wellbeing. You probably know from experience how being stressed, upset or anxious can affect your digestive system. The latest research shows that your brain and digestive system "talk" to each other.

An article on food and mood in the medical journal the BMJ[176] says that to benefit your mood you should be eating a Mediterranean diet or another healthy diet. The Mediterranean diet is rich in fruit, vegetables, fibre and olive oil. It also minimises sugar, processed food and meat.

The researchers say the effect is likely to come about because this diet stabilises blood sugar, encourages a healthy gut microbiome and reduces inflammation. Low level chronic inflammation has been shown to affect the brain as well as the rest of the body.

David Sack MD writing in Psychology Today[177] says:

"The roller coaster of high blood sugar followed by a crash may accentuate the symptoms of mood disorders. Research has tied heavy sugar consumption to an increased risk of depression and worse outcomes in individuals with schizophrenia. There are a couple [of] theories explaining the link. For starters, sugar suppresses activity of a hormone called BDNF which is low in individuals with depression and schizophrenia. Sugar is also at the root of chronic inflammation, which impacts the immune system, the brain, and other systems in the body; inflammation has also been implicated in depression. Interestingly, countries with high sugar intake also have a high rate of depression."

Many people think a diet without many of the things they enjoy will make them miserable. In the short run this may be true, but if you persevere these mood-enhancing changes will almost certainly start to happen. And do remember that the eating patterns recommended for an improved mood are also the eating patterns recommended for warding off the chronic diseases of old age.

Can you learn to be happy?

There's a really interesting article by Richard Davidson[178], who is the founder and chair of the Center for Investigating Healthy Minds at the University of Wisconsin, USA. In it, he says:

"There's no question that certain genetic propensities provide some broad constraints [on our emotions]. But within those broad constraints, there's a huge amount that each of us does that will influence our level of happiness and well-being."

He goes on to say, and I think this is particularly interesting:

"These days I talk about happiness and well-being as being skills. And we don't normally think of them as skills, but there's fundamentally no difference between well-being and learning to play a musical instrument. If you practice, you'll get better. All of my work is pointing in that direction. These days, I talk about happiness and well-being as being skills."

He's saying that you can learn to be happy, just as you can learn to play bridge or learn how to post cat videos on Instagram.

Happiness and exercise

The Victoria State government (Australia)[179] website explains the link between exercise and mental wellbeing:

1. The levels of chemicals in the brain, such as serotonin, stress hormones and endorphins, change in a positive way when you exercise

2. Regular exercise can help you sleep better.

3. Exercise can improve your sense of control, coping ability and self-esteem.

4. Exercise can distract you from negative thoughts and provide opportunities to try new experiences.

5. If you exercise with a group, it can be socially supportive.

6. Exercise increases your energy levels.

7. Physical activity can be an outlet for your frustrations.

8. Exercise can reduce skeletal muscle tension, which helps you feel more relaxed.

It can be hard to get out and do it when you're feeling low. So, it's important to remind yourself of these positive benefits that exercise can give you.

Researchers from McMaster University[180] (Canada) have shown that physical activity may help to 'turn on' genes within skeletal muscles. This can then influence the key metabolic pathways that ultimately promote mood-enhancing chemicals within the brain, which help you to feel happy.

Keeping your skeletal muscles strong helps to boost levels of the feel-good chemical serotonin, for example.

For the study, a group of healthy men, aged 65 and over, followed a 12-week programme of high-intensity interval training (HIIT) on a stationary bike once a week and a strength training session once a fortnight.

Researchers analysed blood samples and changes to muscle and determined that three months of exercise was enough to enhance gene expression within the skeletal muscle.

Dr David Allison, lead author of the study, said:

"Even individuals who are already metabolically healthy - with good weight, good blood pressure and blood sugar levels - need to prioritize regular physical activity to maintain or improve upon their mental health ... We have shown such benefits are still achievable in old age and further emphasize the importance of maintaining an active lifestyle."

Jasper Smits[181], director of the Anxiety Research and Treatment Program at Southern Methodist University in Dallas, USA reviewed research and wrote:

"A bad mood is no longer a barrier to exercise; it is the very reason to exercise."

Happiness and values

Your values are the things you believe are important in the way you live. Possible values include contribution, devoutness, discipline, leadership, loyalty, independence, trustworthiness and usefulness, but there are many more.

For example, if you highly value family, do you spend time with your family? Do you try to understand the point of view of other family members? Do you try to include all your family members in activities?

If you highly value personal independence, do you look after your body and mind so you can stay independent?

If you're not sure of what your values are, find a list of them. It's easy to do that on the internet. Once you have a list, identify the five that are most important to you. Then spend time regularly checking whether you are living by your values.

This is important because in general people are happiest when they are living according to values that matter to them. It's also important you feel good about your values. The MindTools website[182] has an interesting article about values and suggests you ask yourself these questions:

- Do these values make you feel good about yourself?

- Are you proud of your top three values?

- Would you be comfortable and proud to tell your values to people you respect and admire?

- Do these values represent things you would support, even if your choice isn't popular, and it puts you in the minority?

Taking delight in small things

You almost certainly have some small things that are guaranteed to make you happy. What that is may be peculiar to you, but here are some possibilities:

- Completing a daily puzzle faster than you normally do

- The smell of clean laundry

- The colour blue

- The downy hair on your grandchild's arm

- Chopping onions finely

- A particular piece of music

Many people belittle themselves for getting immense satisfaction from small things. You hear people say things like:

"I know it's sad but I get such a lot of satisfaction from ...".

The usual implication is that it's not a good thing to get satisfaction from small things. It shows a slightly shameful side to your character. Maybe it means you're shallow or not very intelligent. But think about this again. Isn't it better to have small things that can give you a sense of happiness and satisfaction, rather than insisting on the big things? Focusing on achieving happiness in small things doesn't mean you can't achieve the big and dramatic things too. Having small go-to things that can make you happy is one of the keys to a happier life.

Make unhappiness harder to achieve

Many people need everything to be right in order to be happy, and only need one thing to go wrong in order to be unhappy. This makes happiness almost unachievable.

Interestingly, there are many more negative words for emotions than positive ones in English.

When things go wrong, remind yourself about all the things that are right in your life. They are still there – focus is what counts. Also think about what having the problem means. Here are some examples, of how you can reframe experiences:

- Too much housework? You could be living in a small one-room shack or on the street without much or even any housework to do.

- Queuing at the supermarket? Look at your groceries – would you prefer not to have money to buy food?

- Sat in a traffic queue? You have a car.

- An untidy house. You have lots of possessions.

- There's nothing on the TV worth watching. You have a TV and you are not blind.

Sometimes catastrophic events do happen and then being unhappy is part of the process. But unhappiness can be self-indulgent, representing a belief that everything should be good and easy for you. Remember what Friedrich Nietzsche said:

"That which does not kill us makes us stronger. "

Mindfulness

Mindfulness is deservedly popular as a way of improving well-being. Mindfulness is a way of learning to stay in the present rather than going over old problems or worrying about the future. You may be anxious or fearful about the past or the future, but will worrying make a difference? Knowing that it won't is one thing, applying it is more difficult. This is where mindfulness comes in. Practising mindfulness teaches you to recognise when you're unhelpfully worrying and bring your thoughts back to the present. You can buy books on mindfulness or do a web search. There are lots of apps available too. I particularly like the Headspace app[183] and the Waking Up app[184].

Cognitive Behavioural Therapy (CBT)

Working with a cognitive behavioural therapist can be very helpful if you can't get rid of persistent negative thoughts or find you are always assuming the worst in a situation. The therapist will work with you to change thoughts, beliefs, and attitudes that aren't helpful. CBT is a solution-focussed approach. It's not looking back in your life to understand why you have these thoughts and beliefs. It's looking to change how you feel and act going forward.

For example, you see someone you know, and you feel they have snubbed you. You're upset and can't decide whether to cut them out of your life or phone them in a panic to ask them why they ignored you. Using CBT, you might ask yourself whether there are other interpretations of this event. An obvious one is that your friend just didn't see you because they were deep in thought. This can help you feel less stressed about the event. You may decide to phone them, but you are likely to be less accusing and upset when you speak to them.

Learning to apply these sorts of strategies to your thoughts can be extremely helpful. Many people find these strategies really useful in relieving anxiety and improving general mental wellbeing.

Other happiness help

If you still find happiness difficult, you may need some help.

Many therapists – counsellors, hypnotherapists, kinesiologists, etc. – can help you deal with upsetting experiences from your past or in the present time.

The Mayo clinic[185] say that Vitamin B-12 and other B vitamins play a role in producing brain chemicals that affect mood and other brain functions. Low levels of B-12 and other B vitamins such as vitamin B-6 and folate may be linked to depression.

Flower remedies work well for many people. These are safe to take, even if you are taking medication. If you search for "flower remedies" on the internet you will find lots of information about them.

Sense of purpose

Growing research indicates that your sense of purpose may help protect you against some of the chronic diseases of old age.

Some people have a strong sense of purpose. They have a clear sense of direction and goals in their life. They see the future as giving them the opportunity to fulfil these goals. If you're one of these people, you are less likely to suffer from cardiovascular disease or cognitive decline.

Researchers[186] even found that a sense of purpose can protect against death from any cause. They assessed self-reported sense of purpose among more than 13,000 people. The results showed that people with the highest sense of purpose indicated the lowest risk of death (15.2 percent mortality risk), compared to people with the lowest sense of purpose (36.5 percent mortality risk).

It's thought that the main reason for this is that those with a sense of purpose are more likely to work harder to stay healthy and well. They are more likely to seek help if they have problems. They want to stay well to achieve their purpose. They believe their lives matter.

Sadly, as people get older, they often feel that making new goals or having a strong sense of purpose is pointless. Yet most people do not know how many years they still have to live. Working with goals and purpose can help give meaning to your life. It can also mean you have a healthier old age.

I've suggested various strategies to help you feel happier. Find one (or two) that feel most relevant and try those.

Loneliness & community

A t one time researchers only looked for physical causes for physical illnesses. Over the years that idea has been recognised as too simple. Researchers have discovered that your mental health can affect your physical health in many different ways.

In recent years the roles that loneliness and lack of purpose play in causing physical and mental ill health has been more understood. Feeling connected and part of a community is now seen as powerful preventive medicine.

Vivek Murthy (19th Surgeon General of the United States) said:

"I trained in internal medicine, and I expected most of my time would be spent on diabetes or heart disease or cancer. What I didn't expect was that so many people I saw would be struggling with loneliness."

The UK charity Campaign To End Loneliness[187] summarises the research on the detrimental health effects of loneliness. Loneliness increases the likelihood of mortality by 26%. This is similar to the impact of being obese or smoking cigarettes. It is also associated with an increased risk of developing high blood pressure, coronary heart disease and stroke. Lonely people become frailer faster than older people who aren't lonely. Loneliness puts individuals at greater risk of depression, cognitive decline and dementia.

The National Institute on Aging[188] (USA) agrees:

"Research has linked social isolation and loneliness to higher risks for a variety of physical and mental conditions: high blood pressure, heart disease, obesity, a weakened immune system, anxiety, depression, cognitive decline, Alzheimer's disease, and even death."

It's not clear yet why loneliness has this effect. It has been suggested that it may be because people are more likely to engage in healthy activities or seek timely medical advice if they are happy and engaged with others. Lonely unhappy people may well feel that there is no point trying to help themselves through eating well, exercising and seeking medical advice. They may feel hopeless.

Family relationships

An Australian study[189] examined data from almost 8,000 women who were free from 11 common long-term conditions and aged 45 to 50 when the study began in 1996. Every three years they reported their satisfaction levels with their partners, family members, friends and work colleagues.

They were tracked for 20 years to see if they developed diabetes, hypertension, heart disease, stroke, chronic obstructive pulmonary disease, asthma, osteoporosis, arthritis, cancer, depression or anxiety.

Those who reported the lowest level of satisfaction with their social relationships had double the risk of developing multiple conditions compared with those who reported the highest levels of satisfaction.

Working to improve these relationships can lead to greater happiness for yourself and for others. It can also mean you are likely to be healthier and less troubled by chronic diseases.

Social activity and art

Paula Gardner[190] of McMaster University, Canada says:

"Staying engaged in activities with friends and community members is key to aging well. Research also suggests that art stimulates us in unique ways, bringing both cognitive and mood benefits. Exercise, art and engagement appear to work synergistically. Together, it's a cocktail for health!"

Caring for a family member

Caring for a family member can have an impact on your experience of loneliness. Researchers[191] looked at 28 studies and found that caring for a partner with complex health conditions, particularly dementia or Alzheimer's disease, is related to higher levels of loneliness. Caring for grandchildren (or other unrelated children) was linked with lower levels of loneliness.

You may not have a choice about caring for a family member. If you are caring for an ill partner, look at ways you can get additional support. Be prepared to ask others for help. You have a right to look after your own health and well-being. If you are feeling lonely, you are likely to become resentful of the other person no matter how much you love them. At the very least, look for support to minimise this resentment and its effect on your loved one.

Loneliness as you age

As you age, it can be difficult to maintain your friendship circle. The potential for meeting new people can be reduced if you stop going out to work. Sadly, some of your friends will die, or they may move away. Because loneliness has a huge effect on both our physical and mental health, you need to work out how to make new friends as you get older.

Many people worry about how they will talk to new people. Starting a conversation is simple – you just say hello! People get anxious and overthink how to approach others or strike up a conversation. Once you've said hello, and they have hopefully responded, tell them your name and ask them theirs, if that's appropriate. Then ask them a simple question about themselves. People love talking about themselves. If you show genuine warmth and curiosity about them, people will usually respond positively.

If all this seems daunting, practise first in situations where it is unimportant – standing in a queue in a supermarket, for example, or waiting for a bus. Here you have readily available topics of conversation to help things along – the price of food, the fact the buses don't run to the timetable. (You probably wouldn't ask them their name though.) It won't always work. You will sometimes be rebuffed, but just keep doing it. You will sometimes have very interesting conversations, and you might just meet your new best friend. At the minimum, you will get practice at how to talk to people you don't know.

You may have lost confidence or never had it. If you concentrate on yourself and how nervous you feel, you may find it difficult to make the first move with a new person. You may appear standoffish and uninterested. So, try and focus on the other people. Remind yourself that they may also be feeling nervous and uncertain.

And do remember that there will be many other people in the same position as you – looking to make new friends. Rather than just focusing on your need for new friends, think about how other people are looking for a friend just like you. They may have moved to a new area, or maybe their best friend or partner has died.

The frequent advice about joining clubs and other sociable events can seem trite, but it's so often offered as at least part of a solution for loneliness because it works.

Introduce your friends to each other. Research shows you feel more supported if your friends know each other. Researcher David Lee[192] of Ohio State University (USA) says:

"The more cohesive, the more dense this network you have, the more you feel you can rely on them for support. It matters if your friends can depend on each other, just like you depend on them.

"People who feel they have more social support in their lives may be focusing more on the collective support they feel from being part of a strong, cohesive group. It's having a real crew, as opposed to just having a set of friends."

Volunteer for longevity and happiness

Volunteering can also be a great way to meet other people. Volunteer in a local charity/thrift shop – they usually have suitable roles even if you don't want to meet the public or operate a pay point. Maybe you could do admin tasks for a charity or do research for a campaigning organisation. Could you help out at a community event?

You may be fearful of joining these sorts of events and organisations but do remember that most of the other people will be there for precisely the same reason: they want to make new friends too.

Older people who volunteer are happier and healthier, so they are less likely to be depressed. It seems obvious when you think about it – volunteering means you are meeting new people, possibly learning new skills and feeling valued and needed.

A 2014 research project[193] confirms all this. The researchers reviewed 73 studies published over the last 45 years involving adults aged 50-plus who were in formal volunteering roles.

The review found that volunteering is associated with reductions in symptoms of depression and better overall health. Volunteers were also living longer than those who didn't volunteer.

They found that you need to volunteer for 2-3 hours per week to feel the benefit. Volunteering for more hours didn't increase these benefits but may still be what you want to do.

If you've got a chronic health condition you may feel volunteering isn't for you, but the research found that people like you benefited the most from volunteering.

Protesting

You can dedicate your life to a cause you care passionately about. Brigit Bardot was a French film actress who became an international sex symbol in the 1950s and '60s. Many people in her position would feel very stressed and depressed by getting older. But she has said:

"I don't feel old or used up, and I don't have time to waste thinking about aging, because I live only for my cause."

When you think of protesters, you may think of teenagers such as Greta Thunberg, or maybe students in their twenties and thirties. You probably don't think of older people taking to the streets and joining protests around the world.

Kuhn, a social activist from the USA, who died when she was 90, said:

"Old age is an excellent time for outrage. My goal is to say or do at least one outrageous thing every week."

In 2004, while I was on holiday in the USA, I met a woman in her seventies. She spent most of her time attending rallies against the then president, George W Bush. I asked her about her energetic activism. She explained that she lived on her own. Her children were grown up and independent. Nobody depended on her, so she felt it didn't matter to anyone else if she were jailed. She was happy taking that risk. Her activism meant she was an energetic and interesting person to talk to. I still remember her well all these years later.

Frances Crowe is a 98-year-old peace activist and clearly agrees with the woman I met in the US. She led a group of eight pipeline opponents in staging a mock funeral for the fossil fuel age near the site of the Kinder Morgan pipeline extension project in Sandisfield, Massachusetts. Crowe said the only way to bring change is to act, not wait for others. She has said[194]:

"Young people are busy getting an education, getting set up in meaningful employment, and then they are busy raising their families. I think it takes the older people like me to step up and put their bodies in the action."

Do you recoil at the idea of taking political action or might it be something you want to explore more?

Does everyone feel lonely?

It's important to stress that just because you live alone or don't have contact with your family or a wide circle of friends you don't necessarily feel lonely.

Psychologist Lane Beckes[195] (Bradley University, USA) says:

"We absolutely need other people."

But he goes on to say:

"A lot of people can ... live alone and be perfectly fine in part because they do things like they talk to their friends on the phone, they have Zoom conversations, they feel like other people will come to their aid."

The degree of loneliness you experience is a direct result of the mismatch between the amount of contact and interaction you have and the amount you want. If there's a big difference, it is likely to impact your mental and physical health.

I've suggested various ways of counteracting loneliness. I don't expect them all to appeal to you. But it's clear that if you are lonely, finding reliable ways of being less lonely will make you happier and also healthier.

Medicines

E arlier in the book I talked about how many older people were taking medicine. It's now unusual not to be taking regular medication when you are older. A 2018 University of Plymouth[196] (UK) study concluded:

"From major heart surgery to a course of minor drugs, people overestimate the benefits and underestimate the risks of a variety of medical procedures ...".

NHS England[197] say it's not just patients that have this problem:

"Both individuals and clinicians tend to consistently over-estimate the benefits of treatments and under-estimate the harms."

Many doctors seem to assume that their patients won't want to make lifestyle changes, so they prescribe long-term medication without any discussion. It is always worth asking your clinicians if there are lifestyle changes or a dietary approach you could try first.

What medicines are not suitable for older adults?

There are particular considerations about taking drugs as you get older. Older bodies are different from younger bodies.

The US healthinaging.org[198] website says:

"The aging process can affect how the medication is absorbed, used in the body, and exits the body. Changes that decrease your body's ability to break down or remove certain medications from your system may mean that medications can stay in your body longer. So, you may need a lower dose of the medication or a different medication that is safer. In most cases, older adults need lower doses of medications than younger adults."

The website[199] also has a list of medications that should be used with caution or avoided by older people:

- Use with caution non-steroidal anti-inflammatory drugs (NSAIDs)

- Use with caution Digoxin (Lanoxin)

- Avoid some diabetes drugs (glyburide and chlorpropamide)

- Avoid muscle relaxants

- Avoid certain medications used for anxiety and/or insomnia

- Avoid certain anticholinergic drugs

- Avoid the pain reliever meperidine (Demerol)

- If you are NOT being treated for psychosis, use antipsychotic drugs with caution

- Avoid certain over-the-counter products that contain antihistamine

- Avoid oestrogen pills and patches

The website recommends these restrictions because, for example, the medication may affect your kidneys, cause grogginess (so you are more likely to fall) or cause confusion.

Of course, you mustn't just stop taking any of these if you have already been prescribed them. Check with your medical practitioner, but quote the healthinaging.org[200] website (not this book!).

Adverse drug reactions

A research article published in the British Journal of General Practice[201] followed older people for six years. They found that one in four older people
experience adverse drug reactions (ADRs) to medicines prescribed by their
primary care physician during this time. Adverse effects included dry mouth,
ankle swelling, headaches and nausea. Often the adverse effect is mild, but in
some people, it is more severe and may even involve hospital admission. The
medicines most commonly associated with ADRs included those used to treat
high blood pressure and other cardiac conditions, strong painkillers such as
tramadol, and antibiotics such as amoxicillin.

Taking multiple different medicines

Older people tend to take more medication than younger people, resulting
sometimes in dangerous interactions between drugs. This multiple drug use is
known as polypharmacy.

The more medications and other products you are on, the greater the chances
of having a medication interaction between two or more drugs.

In addition, the US healthinaging.org[202] website gives this warning:

"Polypharmacy increases the possibility of a "prescribing cascade." A prescribing cascade is when a side effect of one medication is mistaken for a new
medical condition and is then treated with another medication. This can lead
to being prescribed more medications than you need and also further increases
your risk of having more side effects and continuing the cascade. Therefore, ask
your healthcare provider to review all of your medicines with you. And before
you get a new medicine, ask if one of the medicines you are already taking might
be causing the problem the new medicine is meant to treat."

Medical errors

Healthcare professionals dedicate their lives to keeping patients healthy and safe. But medical errors can happen despite the best intentions.

The startling fact[203] is that "Medical errors are a serious public health problem and a leading cause of death in the United States" and other countries too.

Rachel Ann Elliott and colleagues[204] wrote in the medical journal BMJ Quality & Safety that around 237 million medication errors occur in England each year. Many are not really harmful, but "66 million are potentially clinically significant."

The US singlecare website[205] reports that every year, 7,000-9,000 Americans die as a result of a medication error. They go on to say that about one in five hospital admissions in over-65s are caused by the adverse effects of medicines. "The more pills a person takes, the higher the risk that one or more of these medicines will have an unwanted or harmful effect. "

Types of medical errors

There are two major types of errors:

- Errors of omission. For example, not arranging regular liver function tests for someone taking long-term medication that is known to affect the liver.

- Errors of commission occur as a result of the wrong action taken. Examples include administering a medication to which a patient has a known allergy or not labelling a laboratory specimen that is subsequently ascribed to the wrong patient.

They can occur anywhere in the health care system—-hospitals, clinics, out-patient surgery centres, doctors' offices, nursing homes, pharmacies, and in your own home.

General tips to help protect yourself from medical errors

Because of the level of medical errors, you must take an active part in your treatment and drug regime. Don't just assume that the medical people know best:

- Speak up if you have questions or concerns. You have a right to ask questions of anyone involved in your care.

- Make sure that all health professionals involved in your care have any important health information about you. Do not assume that every-one knows everything about you. Even practitioners you have seen for a long time may not remember everything about you.

- If you have a test done, don't assume that no news is good news. Ask about the results, including what the results mean and if you need additional follow-up care.

- Clearly identify yourself to your providers. If you are issued an identi-fication band, keep it on. If you have difficulty hearing, tell the person that you have difficulty hearing. Double-check that it is your name being called. If you have a common name, ask to have the birth date checked in the record to reduce the chance of mistaken identity.

How to avoid drug errors

It's important to be vigilant to prevent medication errors.

- Tell your doctor, pharmacist and nurse about everything you take.

This includes prescription medicines, over-the-counter medicines, and dietary supplements such as vitamins, herbs or other alternative therapies.

- At least once a year, bring all of your medicines and supplements with you to your doctor, nurse or pharmacist and ask them to evaluate them. Have them list all of this in your records.

- Tell your doctor and pharmacist when you start or stop taking any new medications, vitamins, herbs or other therapies so they can check for drug interactions.

- Tell your doctor, pharmacist or nurse about any allergies or adverse reactions you have had to medicines, herbs, chemicals or foods.

- Take a list of everything you are taking when you have a medical visit.

- Instead of relying on your memory, ask (if necessary) for printed information about the side effects and drug interactions that your medicine could cause, as well as printed directions for taking the medicines.

- When you pick up your medicine from the pharmacy, make sure it is the medicine you've been prescribed. If the medicine is one that you have been taking and it looks different, ask the pharmacist to double-check before taking the drug.

- Be sure you understand the directions on your medicine label. For example, ask if "four doses daily" means taking a dose every 6 hours around the clock or just during regular waking hours.

- Ask your pharmacist for the best device to measure liquid medicine. Household teaspoons often do not hold a true teaspoon of liquid, so use specially marked syringes or measuring spoons to measure the right dose.

- If the medicine requires a special device (for example, an inhaler), be sure you understand how to use it correctly. Practice in front of your care provider to demonstrate that you are using the device properly.

Ask questions about your medication

Ask for information about your medicines in terms you can understand. You have a right to know. Here are some possible questions:

- What is this medicine for?

- How am I supposed to take it and for how long?

- Is this medicine safe to take with other medicines, herbs or dietary supplements?

- What food, drink, or activities should I avoid while taking this medicine?

- What side effects are likely?

- What do I do if they occur?

You are likely to forget up to 80% of what your doctor tells you!

A study published in the Journal of the Royal Society of Medicine[206] found that most patients forget as much as 80 percent of what their doctor tells them as soon as they leave the clinic. The study was published in 2003, but the results are unlikely to have changed.

Study author Dr. Roy Kessels explains why patients forget crucial medical information:

"Memory for medical information is often poor and inaccurate, especially when the patient is old or anxious. Patients tend to focus on diagnosis-related information and fail to register instructions on treatment."

Food and drug interaction

Some foods affect drug absorption and use. This is usually set out in the leaflet that comes with the drug, so make sure you read the leaflet. Examples include:

- Garlic can affect anticoagulants and diabetes medication.

- Grapefruit can cause the body to absorb more of some drugs such as antihistamines, statins, benzodiazepines and anti-anxiety medication such as buspirone.

- Alcohol interacts with some drugs particularly those that have an effect on the brain, e.g. sleeping pills, antidepressants.

- Over-ripe cheese, pickles, some beers and red wine can affect MAOI antidepressants, leading to a dangerous rise in blood pressure.

- Cranberry juice can affect Warfarin.

- Salty foods and liquid can affect lithium.

- St John's Wort (a supplement) may affect the contraceptive pill and the antidepressant Prozac.

- Ginkgo biloba (a supplement) can affect anticoagulants.

This is not a completely comprehensive list, so always ask your doctor and check the leaflet that comes with your medicines.

Effect of drugs in nutritional terms

Drugs can affect your absorption of nutrition from your food in several different ways.

Some drugs cause gastric irritation, (e.g., aspirin and non-steroidal anti-inflammatory drugs). These should be taken with food to minimise this problem.

Some drugs change gastrointestinal pH. For example, antacids neutralise stomach acids and so reduce vitamin B12 absorption.

Some drugs change gastrointestinal motility, particularly laxatives. 'Gastrointestinal motility' is the medical term for how fast food moves through the stomach and intestine. If food moves more quickly through the intestine, it may be difficult for the body to extract all the nutrients it needs. Aluminium, which is in many antacids, has a relaxing effect on some muscles and so slows the process down – good for nutrient absorption, but it can cause constipation.

Some drugs form insoluble complexes with components of food. This means that neither the drug nor the nutrient (usually a mineral) will be absorbed. For example, tetracyclines bind to calcium in dairy products.

Some drugs affect nutrient metabolism and distribution. For example, anti-convulsive drugs affect folic acid metabolism. Aspirin competes with folate for binding sites on serum proteins.

Some drugs affect nutrient excretion, causing more or less of a particular nutrient to be excreted. For example, corticosteroids increase the excretion of potassium and increase the retention of sodium. Diuretics may increase the excretion of potassium, magnesium, calcium and the water-soluble B vitamins and vitamin C.

Some drugs affect the bowel flora. Your intestine contains millions of useful bacteria that produce some vitamins and contribute to proper digestion and a healthy immune system. There are also other harmful bacteria that can compete with the good bacteria. Antibiotics lead to a reduction of the beneficial bacteria.

If you have been taking antibiotics, I strongly recommend you take a probiotic supplement to repopulate your gut with healthy bacteria.

Some drugs can lead to changes in appetite. For example, anti-convulsant drugs can cause diarrhoea and reduce appetite.

Steroid drugs have the potential to interfere with the absorption and utilisation of calcium, potassium, sodium, protein, and vitamins C and D. Aspirin has been reported to lower plasma vitamin C concentrations, but how it does this is not known.

Certain drugs (metformin, proton pump inhibitors) can reduce absorption of B12, so you may need to talk to your doctor about taking a supplement.

Statins

More than 40 million Americans take statins, the most common type of prescription drug. While statins have been shown to effectively lower cholesterol levels and reduce the risks of stroke and heart attack, they do not work the same for everyone, and side effects of statin use include an increased risk of developing type 2 diabetes. There is some evidence[207] that the gut microbiome affects a person's reactions to statins, but that work is still at an early stage.

Many patients have reported that statins cause muscle pain or weakness. A study published in the medical journal The Lancet[208] looked at data on 155,000 patients from 23 trials of statins. The researchers found that when a patient reported muscle symptoms while taking a statin, there was a less than 10% chance that the pain was caused by the drug. They also suggested that the small increased risk of muscle symptoms was mostly observed within the first year of treatment.

The Oxford researchers stressed that if patients experienced muscle symptoms they should tell their GP. They also acknowledged that in very rare cases the drug can cause quite serious muscle damage.

People taking statins may also develop type 2 diabetes. The Mayo Clinic says:

"It's possible your blood sugar (blood glucose) level may increase when you take a statin, which may lead to developing type 2 diabetes. The risk is small but important enough that the Food and Drug Administration (FDA) has issued a warning on statin labels regarding blood glucose levels and diabetes.

"The increase generally occurs when blood sugar levels are already higher than normal and fall in the prediabetes or diabetes range when you begin taking a statin."

This possibility is something to be aware of. You need to consult your health professional if you think this is happening to you.

Supplements

The US National Institute on Aging website[209] says this:

"People over age 50 may need more of some vitamins and minerals than younger adults do. Your doctor or a dietitian can tell you whether you need to change your diet or take a vitamin or mineral supplement to get enough of these."

The website explains the possible problems – shortage of calcium, vitamin D, vitamin B6 and vitamin B12.

The Dietary Guidelines for Americans, 2020-2025[210] (a PDF not a web page)) recommends how much of each vitamin and mineral men and women of different ages need. For example:

"**Vitamin B12**: 2.4 mcg (micrograms) each day. If you are taking medicine for acid reflux, you might need a different form, which your healthcare provider can give you information about.

"**Calcium**: Women over age 50 need 1,200 mg (milligrams) each day. Men need 1,000 mg between age 51 and 70 and 1,200 mg after 70, but not more than 2,000 mg a day.

"**Vitamin D**: 600 IU (International Units) for people aged 51 to 70, and 800 IU for those over 70, but not more than 4,000 IU each day.

"**Vitamin B6**: 1.7 mg for men and 1.5 mg for women each day."

The website goes on to say:

"Sometimes, too much of a vitamin or mineral can be harmful. Most if not all of your daily vitamins and minerals should come from food. When thinking about whether you need more of a vitamin or mineral, think about how much of each nutrient you get from food and drinks, as well as from any supplements you take."

This information is for guidance. It is definitely best to consult your doctor or some properly qualified health adviser.

Vitamin B12

Vitamin B12 is an important vitamin. Many people know that vegans need to take a vitamin B supplement to stay healthy, but what about everyone else?

Diane Cress[211], Associate Professor of Nutrition and Food Science, Wayne State University, says:

"One primary symptom of B12 deficiency is fatigue – a level of tiredness or exhaustion so deep that it affects daily life activities.

"Other symptoms are neurological and may include tingling in the extremities, confusion, memory loss, depression and difficulty maintaining balance. Some of these can be permanent if the vitamin deficiency is not addressed.

"However, since there can be so many causes for these symptoms, health care providers may overlook the possibility of a B12 deficiency and fail to screen for it."

The absorption of B12 from your food is a complex process. If you suffer from a dry mouth because of medication, your body may struggle to absorb the B12 in your diet. Low stomach acid is common as you age. This can also make absorption difficult. The drug Metformin, used to treat Type 2 diabetes, has been associated with B12 deficiency for decades.

So, if you are experiencing any of these symptoms it may be a good idea to ask your health care provider to check for a B12 deficiency. This is particularly true if you have a dry mouth, take Metformin or have low stomach acid.

Vitamin D

Vitamin D is required for the proper use of calcium and phosphorus in the body. That makes it essential for the maintenance of musculoskeletal health. Any deficiency could result in bone deformities such as osteomalacia in adults.

Sunlight is an excellent source of vitamin D. In some countries where sunlight is limited in the winter vitamin D supplements are recommended for all adults at that time of the year. In the UK a daily supplement containing 10 micrograms of vitamin D is recommended from October to March.

If you live somewhere that is generally sunnier than the UK, you may only need a vitamin D supplement if you spend all or most of your time indoors. If you have a dark skin, your body will produce less vitamin D, so supplementation may be advisable. If you normally cover most of your skin when you are outdoors, supplementation is also recommended.

Aids & comfort

As people get older, they often turn to various appliances to make their life easier. They may even move to an apartment or bungalow to avoid having to walk upstairs.

Riser recliner chairs make it easier to stand and sit safely. Walking sticks and walking frames can help frail people to move around more safely. Older people often put chairs and stools in strategic places to minimise the amount of standing they need to do. For example, a stool in the bathroom can allow them to clean their teeth or shave while sitting down.

These and other aids and changes can allow people to stay independent for longer and ease some of the burden of old age that they feel.

At first sight, these adaptations seem completely positive, but there is also a downside to all this.

Research shows that stair climbing is beneficial. Dr. Sophie Paddock[212] of the University of East Anglia (UK) looked at the research on stair climbing. She reviewed studies that in total included over 480,000 participants. She concluded:

"Based on these results, we would encourage people to incorporate stair climbing into their day-to-day lives. Our study suggested that the more stairs climbed, the greater the benefits [for heart health]."

Duke Human Resources website[213] from Duke University (USA) has set up "Take the Stairs, a stair-stepping program that can help you increase your physical activity, get closer to your health goals, and earn prizes." Check out their website for more details about the program and the prizes.

They list these benefits of stair climbing:

- A significantly lower risk of mortality when climbing more than 55 flights per week.

- Stair climbing requires about 8 - 11kcal of energy per minute, which is high compared to other moderate level physical activities.

- Active stair climbers are more fit and have a higher aerobic capacity.

- Even two flights of stairs climbed each day can lead to 6 lbs of weight loss over one year.

- There is a strong association between stair climbing and bone density in post-menopausal women.

- Climbing stairs can improve the amount of "good cholesterol" in the blood.

- Stair climbing increases leg power and may be an important priority in reducing the risk of injury from falls in the elderly.

- Stair climbing can help you build and maintain healthy bones, muscles and joints.

Reducing the amount you stand may not be a good idea either. A study published in the Journal of Science and Medicine in Sport[214] looked at 64 sedentary middle-aged adults with metabolic syndrome. Half the group was told to maintain their normal habits. The others were instructed to increase standing and light-intensity physical activity by one hour per day, although most managed only 50 minutes. This group had "beneficial effects in several cardiometabolic risk markers" after three months. So, think before you make life easier for yourself with those additional chairs.

I recently spoke to John Gullick. John is a health coach with a background in physiotherapy. You can see my interview with him on YouTube[215]. John says:

"To become supple, interact with hard surfaces. To become stiff, interact with soft surfaces."

When you sit in a comfortable chair, your body doesn't prompt you to keep moving. You may feel stiff from this lack of movement when you get up. You may blame the chair. In a way that's true, but it's because it is too comfortable. It's not uncomfortable enough to keep you making slight adjustments all the time.

John also says:

"The best posture is the next one: we need movement, not "optimal" static positions. These basically don't exist."

It's a fine balance between finding aids that help keep you active and independent, and aids that stop you exercising properly, leading to declining health. I don't have a magic formula for deciding this. Recognising the possibility that aids can increase your frailty will hopefully lead you to examine your options more carefully.

Achieving your goals

I hope that reading this book will inspire you to make some lifestyle changes. But sadly, for many people good intentions don't readily promote consistent meaningful actions. Psychologists call this the intention-behaviour gap.

I suggest you start small. Go for one or two goals and get them embedded in your life so they become normal for you. Then add more.

If you decide to start going to the gym, switch to a wholefood plant-based diet and start volunteering for a local homeless charity, you are unlikely to do any of them consistently.

Apart from starting small, what else can you do?

Sleep well to achieve your goals

A study[216] supported by the American Heart Association found that participants who reported getting regular, uninterrupted sleep did a better job sticking to their exercise and diet plans while trying to lose weight. This is perhaps not a surprising result, but it probably underlines your own experience that when you haven't slept well, you are likely to make poor decisions.

Colin Chapman[217], Uppsala University (Sweden) and colleagues found that people who were deprived of one night's sleep purchased more food (in terms of calories and weight) in a mock supermarket the following day.

If you often don't sleep well, check out the practical suggestions in the Sleep chapter.

Making healthy behaviours part of your identity

Do you have a self-identity that includes eating healthily at least most of the time, caring about your community, taking exercise, or doing any of the other positive actions in this book? If you do, you are more likely consistently to follow through. It becomes less hard to exert self-control and be consistent. Positive affirmations can help. Writing in a journal each day, reflecting on your emotions, your behaviour and your goals can be very helpful too.

Sharing your goals with others

How many times have you seen the advice that you should share your goals? The theory is that it increases your accountability, and success comes with accountability.

But research suggests that this is not always correct. In fact, research suggests that you are likely to be less successful if you share your goals. Research says that you should keep your goals to yourself.

A study[218] by psychologist Peter Gollwitzer and colleagues of New York University (USA) looked at study goals for students. In the results of this study and subsequent studies performed on other students, the experimenters found that the students whose intentions were known tended to act less on their intentions than those whose intentions were unknown. When the students kept their study goals to themselves, they were more likely to achieve them.

The researchers concluded that telling people what you want to achieve creates a premature sense of completeness. While you feel a sense of pride in letting people know what you intend to do, that pride doesn't motivate you and can in fact hurt you later.

Another study[219] analysed data from 364 clients who signed up for an online weight management service. In the trial clients voluntarily completed a baseline survey and then were randomly assigned to one of three different groups.

The first group had to nominate a friend or family member to keep track of whether they had met their weight loss commitment.

The second group was offered a refund on their subscription, regardless of whether they met their target weight in the coming weeks.

The third group – the comparison group - were clients who continued to pay the monthly fee, so maintained a financial commitment to achieve their weight loss target.

The study measured weight loss outcomes at 12 weeks and found that on average all participants lost weight. The refund group lost 2.4% on average and the comparison group lost on average 2.2% of initial body weight.

The group that was asked to share their goals with friends or family reported the slowest rate of weight loss with an average of 1.1%. They lost approximately half of what the other two groups lost.

This is the opposite of what you would expect from all that advice about sharing goals to increase accountability. The researchers are not totally certain why this is so.

Think carefully before you share goals with others. Don't assume it is going to help.

Commit to behaviour as well as goals

It's important to have goals, but it's also important to set behaviour intentions. When I concentrate on my behaviour rather than fretting about outcomes, I achieve more with less stress. I can let the goal take care of itself. My behaviour is what counts. Here are some behaviour-focussed commitments to get you started:

- I'll do a mindfulness mediation every weekday.

- I'll plan and prep three healthy meals on a Monday to eat during the rest of the week.

- I'll go the gym for at least 40 minutes on Monday, Wednesday and Friday.

I'm not committing to a goal or outcome; I am committing to a process. I know that if I follow through on the process, I'm likely to achieve more and, crucially, with much less stress.

Implementation intentions

"Implementation intentions" are what psychologists call "if-then" plans. This is where you plan what you will do in challenging situations. You don't just hope the challenge won't happen.

Here are some examples:

- If Mary insists on giving me a box of chocolates, I'll thank her and give it secretly to a foodbank.

- If I'm within 200 steps of my goal for the day, I'll walk round the house till I reach it.

- If I have a really bad day with eating, I'll focus on eating extra fibre the next day.

- If my mother tells me all this exercise will be bad for my back, I'll quote the research that shows it helps chronic back pain. I'll also thank her for her concern.

You may want to have more than one alternative strategy. For example:

"If people press me to drink more alcohol at the next big family party, I'll offer to get them a drink without getting one for myself. Alternatively, I'll say that I think I've discovered I may be allergic to it. If that doesn't seem appropriate, I'll accept the drink and then find a way to pour it away without anyone knowing."

Here you have three options. Hopefully one of them will be easy to implement.

Get the idea? None of these situations may be ones you are likely to encounter but think about what the obstacles are likely to be for you. Then make an if-then plan.

Monitor your progress

People who want to lose weight and keep it off usually benefit from weighing themselves regularly. This can be every day or every week, so you would need to find what works for you.

There are various apps that will allow you to track your progress in losing weight, taking exercise or sleeping more soundly. Many people find these very helpful.

You can also use an Excel spreadsheet or a paper and pen to monitor your progress too.

Some people find monitoring their progress in this way leads to a lot of self-criticism or obsessive behaviour. If that happens to you, this may not be a useful thing to do.

Motivate yourself

Remember the carrot-and-stick of traditional thinking? It still has relevance today.

Think about the past: what motivated you to do things you didn't want to do or that were difficult? These don't have to be major goals, just tasks that you managed to complete despite yourself.

Did you plan to reward yourself when you completed the task? Did you think about the satisfaction you would feel when you achieved your goal? Did you think about how other people would be pleased or impressed? If these or similar approaches got you going, you are motivated by the 'carrot'. You are motivated by the positive outcomes.

Did you think about the disappointment you would feel if you didn't succeed? Did you think about other people's disapproval? Did you deny yourself something until you completed your goal? If these or similar approaches helped, you are motivated by the 'stick'. You are motivated by negative factors.

Is it sometimes the carrot and sometimes the stick? Can you see a pattern to this? Are work goals usually motivated by the stick, and home goals by the carrot? Do you ever use both at the same time? Spend some time thinking about this, and see what patterns emerge.

Whatever they are, apply this to whatever you want to do. It will help to keep you motivated to achieve your heart's desires. There isn't a wrong or right answer to this - understanding how motivation works for you will help you achieve much more in your life.

Keep trying

Don't give up. When I was in my twenties I was smoking around 40 cigarettes a day. I made numerous attempts to give up smoking before I actually succeeded. The important thing to remember is not to keep trying in exactly the same way each time. Make small changes to find what works for you.

The evidence is there. We know beyond doubt that making positive lifestyle changes can show big benefits whatever your age and state of health.

Books by Jane Thurnell-Read

I'd appreciate it if you took the time to leave a review wherever you bought this book. Reviews help readers see books that would be a good fit for them. They also help me to sell more books.

All books are available on Amazon as eBooks and paperbacks. The first three are also available as audiobooks, via Amazon, Audible and iTunes.

- 190 Weight Loss Hacks: How to lose weight naturally and permanently without stress

- Menopause Weight Loss: Live well, sleep well, stop hot flashes and lose weight

- The Science of Healthy Ageing: Unlocking the Secrets to Longevity, Vitality, and Disease Prevention

Specialist books for CAM therapists

- Energy Mismatch for Kinesiologists, Dowsers & EAV Practitioners

- Verbal Questioning Skills for Kinesiologists & Dowsers

About the author

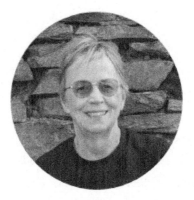

I have been a university lecturer, a complementary therapist and an entrepreneur over the years. But throughout that time, I've loved books and writing. I enjoy sharing difficult information and ideas with others in a way that doesn't dumb it down or disrespect people. People say that's one of my superpowers!

I'm now in my seventies – I'm fit, strong and healthy. That didn't happen by accident. In my twenties, I drank heavily (a quarter of a bottle of whisky a day) and smoked around 40 cigarettes a day. My diet consisted of toast, chocolate and orange juice. I learnt bit by bit how to change that and become happier and healthier.

In my late forties, I learnt to ride a bike. In my sixties, I fell in love with lifting heavy weights in the gym.

I know that small changes can have a big impact on our lives. I believe in sharing practical, research-based information that you can easily apply in your life too.

I want to inspire and inform you, so you can be happier and healthier than you've ever been.

You can connect with me on

Youtube: https://tinyurl.com/yt999-jtr

Instagram @thrivingjane

Website www.janethurnellread.com

1. https://www.ons.gov.uk/peoplepopulationandcommunity/healthandsocialcare/healthandlifeexpectancies/bulletins/healthstatelifeexpectanciesuk/2018to2020

2. https://www.ncoa.org/article/the-top-10-most-common-chronic-conditions-in-older-adults

3. https://www.cdc.gov/chronicdisease/index.htm

4. https://www.canada.ca/en/public-health/services/publications/diseases-conditions/aging-chronic-diseases-profile-canadian-seniors-report.html

5. https://evidence.nihr.ac.uk/alert/multi-morbidity-predicted-to-increase-in-the-uk-over-the-next-20-years/

6. https://www.kff.org/health-reform/issue-brief/data-note-prescription-drugs-and-older-adults/

7. https://academic.oup.com/ageing/article/47/2/220/4237359

8. https://www.mayoclinic.org/diseases-conditions/periodontitis/symptoms-causes/syc-20354473

9. https://www.georgeinstitute.org/media-releases/best-evidence-yet-that-lowering-blood-pressure-can-prevent-dementia

10. https://news.osu.edu/baby-boomers-show-concerning-decline-in-cognitive-functioning/

11. https://evidence.nihr.ac.uk/alert/multi-morbidity-predicted-to-increase-in-the-uk-over-the-next-20-years/

12. https://www.bbc.com/future/article/20220719-can-you-delay-ageing-by-refusing-to-act-your-age

13. https://www.heart.org/en/news/2022/08/19/how-you-feel-about-aging-could-affect-health-heres-how-to-keep-the-right-attitude

14. https://www.heart.org/en/news/2022/08/19/how-you-feel-about-aging-could-affect-health-heres-how-to-keep-the-right-attitude

15. https://pubmed.ncbi.nlm.nih.gov/31289097/

16. https://www.un.org/en/chronicle/article/lifestyle-diseases-economic-burden-health-services

17. https://www.cancerresearchuk.org/health-professional/cancer-statistics/risk

18. https://www.sciencedaily.com/releases/2019/12/191219142739.htm

19. http://www.genesinlife.org/genes-your-health

20. https://news.wsu.edu/press-release/2022/12/06/twin-study-links-exercise-to-beneficial-epigenetic-changes/

21. https://www.sciencedaily.com/releases/2021/08/210826170151.htm

22. https://news.berkeley.edu/2022/10/07/age-vs-genetics-which-is-more-important-for-how-you-age/

23. https://www.cancerresearchuk.org/about-cancer/causes-of-cancer/inherited-cancer-genes-and-increased-cancer-risk/family-history-and-inherited-cancer-genes

24. https://www.wcrf-uk.org/preventing-cancer/what-can-increase-your-risk-of-cancer/inherited-genes-family-history-and-cancer-risk/

25. https://www.sciencedaily.com/releases/2021/07/210728105633.htm

26. https://ucsdnews.ucsd.edu/pressrelease/physical-activity-may-have-a-stronger-role-than-genes-in-longevity

27. https://alz-journals.onlinelibrary.wiley.com/doi/10.1002/alz.12001

28. https://journals.plos.org/plosmedicine/article?id=10.1371/journal.pmed.1003972

29. https://www.ideafit.com/personal-training/overcoming-genetic-predisposition-with-exercise/

30. https://www.aging-us.com/article/202913/text

31. https://www.hopkinsmedicine.org/health/wellness-and-prevention/its-never-too-late-five-healthy-steps-at-any-age

32. https://www.amjmed.com/article/S0002-9343(06)01185-5/fulltext

33. https://www.escardio.org/The-ESC/Press-Office/Press-releases/It-s-never-too-late-to-get-active

34. https://www.ucsf.edu/news/2024/05/427571/prostate-cancer-study-more-health-benefits-plant-based-diet

35. http://158.39.201.81:3838/Food/

36. https://www.sydney.edu.au/news-opinion/news/2022/09/13/pace-as-important-as-10-000-steps-for-health.html

37. https://www.psu.edu/news/research/story/peanuts-and-herbs-and-spices-may-positively-impact-gut-microbiome

38. https://pubmed.ncbi.nlm.nih.gov/19661958/

39. https://www.kcl.ac.uk/news/snacking-on-almonds-boosts-gut-health

40. https://www.psu.edu/news/research/story/peanuts-and-herbs-and-spices-may-positively-impact-gut-microbiome

41. https://www.cuimc.columbia.edu/news/rx-prolonged-sitting-five-minute-stroll-every-half-hour

42. https://www.sydney.edu.au/news-opinion/news/2022/12/09/one-minute-bursts-of-activity-during-daily-tasks-could-prolong-y.html

43. https://www.sciencedaily.com/releases/2019/07/190719173554.htm

44. https://www.un.org/en/chronicle/article/lifestyle-diseases-economic-burden-health-services

45. https://www.sciencedaily.com/releases/2022/04/220428125433.htm

46. https://www.valterlongo.com/daily-longevity-diet-for-adults/

47. https://www.winchesterhospital.org/health-library/article?id=156995

48. https://onlinelibrary.wiley.com/doi/full/10.1111/joim.13333

49. https://pubmed.ncbi.nlm.nih.gov/32658243/

50. https://www.aan.com/PressRoom/Home/PressRelease/4913

51. https://www.heart.org/en/healthy-living/healthy-eating/add-color/eat-more-color

52. https://www.wcrf-uk.org/our-blog/could-you-eat-30-plant-based-foods-each-week/

53. https://www.express.co.uk/life-style/health/1718381/how-to-live-longer-eat-plant-based-diet-reduce-risk-early-death

54. https://www.helpguide.org/articles/healthy-eating/choosing-healthy-fats.htm

55. https://www.mayoclinic.org/healthy-lifestyle/nutrition-and-healthy-eating/expert-answers/cooking-oil/faq-20058170

56. https://www.nutritionletter.tufts.edu/healthy-eating/health-benefits-of-nuts-and-seeds/

57. https://theconversation.com/ultra-processed-foods-its-not-just-their-low-nutritional-value-thats-a-concern-189918

58. https://www.sciencedaily.com/releases/2019/05/190529221040.htm

59. https://www.bmj.com/company/newsroom/new-evidence-links-ultra-processed-foods-with-a-range-of-health-risks/

60. https://www.cambridge.org/core/journals/public-health-nutrition/article/ultraprocessed-family-foods-in-australia-nutrition-claims-health-claims-and-marketing-techniques/BDF0E999C117FEE3DF2CA175C36D250D

61. https://news.wsu.edu/press-release/2022/02/02/more-spice-could-help-seniors-avoid-salt/

62. https://www.who.int/news-room/fact-sheets/detail/salt-reduction

63. https://www.sciencedaily.com/releases/2023/01/230110103453.htm

64. https://www.health.qld.gov.au/news-events/news/6-things-about-salt-that-arent-true

65. https://news.wsu.edu/press-release/2022/02/02/more-spice-could-help-seniors-avoid-salt/

66. https://www.actiononsalt.org.uk/salthealth/salt-and-obesity/

67. https://nutritionfacts.org/video/how-to-treat-asthma-with-a-low-salt-diet/

68. https://www.sciencedaily.com/releases/2019/02/190220145044.htm

69. https://nutritionfacts.org/video/sodium-and-autoimmune-disease-rubbing-salt-in-the-wound/

70. https://www.sciencedaily.com/releases/2019/06/190627143931.htm

71. https://www.heartandstroke.ca/articles/low-salt-shopping

72. https://www.health.harvard.edu/heart-health/the-sweet-danger-of-sugar

73. https://theconversation.com/curious-kids-are-sugar-rushes-real-161494

74. https://www.sciencedaily.com/releases/2020/09/200917180414.htm

75. https://theconversation.com/sugar-isnt-just-empty-fattening-calories-its-making-us-sick-49788

76. https://nutritionfacts.org/video/flashback-friday-effect-of-sucralose-splenda-on-the-microbiome/

77. https://news.umanitoba.ca/artificial-sweeteners-linked-to-risk-of-long-term-weight-gain-heart-disease-and-other-health-issues/

78. https://news.illinois.edu/view/6367/240046

79. https://theconversation.com/sweeteners-may-be-linked-to-increased-cancer-risk-new-research-179709

80. https://www.medicalnewstoday.com/articles/318435

81. https://theconversation.com/sweeteners-may-be-linked-to-increased-cancer-risk-new-research-179709

82. https://www.sciencedaily.com/releases/2022/03/220324143800.htm

83. https://healthcareassociates.com/can-dehydration-cause-high-blood-pressure/

84. https://www.sciencedirect.com/science/article/pii/S1550413123000517?via%3Dihub

85. https://www.aan.com/PressRoom/Home/PressRelease/5048

86. https://www.un.org/en/chronicle/article/lifestyle-diseases-economic-burden-health-services

87. https://theconversation.com/watching-your-weight-you-may-only-need-to-make-small-changes-to-your-daily-routine-197327

88. https://www.pbrc.edu/news/media/2021/metabolism-milestones.aspx

89. https://warwick.ac.uk/newsandevents/pressreleases/age_is_no

90. https://www.bhf.org.uk/informationsupport/heart-matters-magazine/medical/measuring-your-waist

91. https://www.bhf.org.uk/informationsupport/heart-matters-magazine/medical/measuring-your-waist

92. https://geni.us/jtr-hacks

93. https://theconversation.com/older-people-with-alcohol-dependence-problems-desperately-need-better-support-121198

94. https://ccsa.ca/more-6-drinks-week-puts-your-health-risk-new-canadas-guidance-alcohol-and-health

95. https://www.mentalhealth.org.uk/explore-mental-health/a-z-topics/mental-health-later-life

96. https://www.nia.nih.gov/health/facts-about-aging-and-alcohol

97. https://aru.ac.uk/news/14-units-a-week-still-harmful-to-health

98. https://www.nia.nih.gov/health/facts-about-aging-and-alcohol

99. https://alcoholexplained.com/is-red-wine-good-for-you-2/

100. https://www.cdc.gov/alcohol/faqs.htm

101. https://www.un.org/en/chronicle/article/lifestyle-diseases-economic-burden-health-services

102. https://www.cdc.gov/tobacco/quit_smoking/how_to_quit/benefits/index.htm

103. https://www.cdc.gov/cancer/lung/basic_info/risk_factors.htm

104. https://www.sciencedaily.com/releases/2021/01/210121132140.htm

105. https://www.cdc.gov/chronicdisease/resources/publications/factsheets/diabetes-prediabetes.htm

106. https://www.60plus.smokefree.gov/quit-smoking-women/challenges-when-quitting/weight-gain

107. https://www.cdc.gov/tobacco/basic_information/e-cigarettes/Quick-Facts-on-the-Risks-of-E-cigarettes-for-Kids-Teens-and-Young-Adults.html#quitting-vaping

108. https://www.heart.org/en/healthy-living/healthy-lifestyle/quit-smoking-tobacco/the-benefits-of-quitting-smoking-now

109. https://www.gov.uk/government/news/vaping-better-than-nicotine-re placement-therapy-for-stopping-smoking-evidence-suggests

110. https://publichealth.jhu.edu/2019/vaping-q-and-a-hopkins-expert-on -ecigarettes-and-tobacco-alternatives

111. https://hub.jhu.edu/2021/10/07/vaping-unknown-chemicals/

112. https://www.cochranelibrary.com/cdsr/doi/10.1002/14651858.CD01 3229.pub2/full

113. https://www.60plus.smokefree.gov/tools-tips-women/text-programs

114. https://60plus.smokefree.gov/

115. https://smokefree.gov/build-your-quit-plan

116. https://www.un.org/en/chronicle/article/lifestyle-diseases-economic-b urden-health-services

117. https://dailynews.mcmaster.ca/articles/on-international-day-of-older-p ersons-mcmaster-experts-weigh-in-on-what-it-takes-to-age-well/

118. https://www.heart.org/en/healthy-living/fitness/fitness-basics/why-is -physical-activity-so-important-for-health-and-wellbeing

119. https://www.nhs.uk/live-well/exercise/exercise-health-benefits/

120. https://www.sciencedaily.com/releases/2023/03/230322190900.htm

121. https://www.webmd.com/healthy-aging/features/exercise-older-adults

122. https://www.nia.nih.gov/health/exercising-chronic-conditions

123. https://www.webmd.com/healthy-aging/features/exercise-older-adults

124. https://www.who.int/news-room/fact-sheets/detail/physical-activity

125. https://theconversation.com/four-ways-older-adults-can-get-back-to-e xercising-without-the-worry-of-an-injury-164181

126. https://www.ncbi.nlm.nih.gov/pmc/articles/PMC4934575/

127. https://www.heart.org/en/healthy-living/fitness/fitness-basics/aha-recs -for-physical-activity-in-adults

128. https://www.sciencedaily.com/releases/2023/02/230228205249.htm

129. https://www.nytimes.com/2003/03/05/nyregion/for-elderly-fear-of-fa lling-is-a-risk-in-itself.html

130. https://www.gov.uk/government/publications/falls-applying-all-our-h ealth/falls-applying-all-our-health

131. https://www.ncoa.org/news/resources-for-reporters/get-the-facts/falls -prevention-facts/

132. https://www.ncoa.org/article/get-the-facts-on-healthy-aging

133. https://www.nhs.uk/conditions/falls/prevention/

134. https://www.youtube.com/user/physicaltherapyvideo

135. https://www.youtube.com/c/Alyssaadventurealive

136. https://fallsassistant.org.uk/exercise-centre/

137. https://jamanetwork.com/journals/jamanetworkopen/fullarticle/278 3711

138. https://jamanetwork.com/journals/jamainternalmedicine/fullarticle/2 734709

139. https://www.sydney.edu.au/news-opinion/news/2022/09/13/pace-as-important-as-10-000-steps-for-health.html

140. https://www.aarp.org/health/healthy-living/info-2019/nordic-walking.html

141. https://www.bhf.org.uk/informationsupport/heart-matters-magazine/activity/exercises-heart-health

142. https://www.bhf.org.uk/informationsupport/heart-matters-magazine/activity/exercises-heart-health

143. https://www.cdc.gov/physicalactivity/basics/measuring/index.html

144. https://www.ncbi.nlm.nih.gov/pmc/articles/PMC3117172/

145. https://www.unimelb.edu.au/newsroom/news/2021/october/busting-the-slow-down-myth-vigorous-activity-needed-in-later-life-to-live-longer-and-better

146. https://hasfit.com/

147. https://hasfit.com/workouts/home/senior/

148. https://www.ncbi.nlm.nih.gov/pmc/articles/PMC8947639/

149. https://www.nccih.nih.gov/health/tai-chi-what-you-need-to-know#hedl

150. https://www.ed.ac.uk/news/2019/yoga-improves-health-in-later-life-study-says

151. https://newsinhealth.nih.gov/2019/11/yoga-health

152.
https://www.nccih.nih.gov/research/research-results/study-sees-benefici
al-role-of-yoga-in-weight-loss-program-for-adults-with-obesity-or-overwe
ight

153. https://www.amjmed.com/article/S0002-93430501056-9/fulltext

154. https://www.canada.ca/en/public-health/services/publications/diseases
-conditions/aging-chronic-diseases-profile-canadian-seniors-report.html

155. https://www.ucl.ac.uk/news/2022/oct/five-hours-sleep-night-linked-hi
gher-risk-multiple-diseases

156. https://www.mayoclinic.org/diseases-conditions/insomnia/in-depth/sl
eeping-pills/art-20043959

157. https://www.express-scripts.com/pharmacy/blog/medications-that-can
-affect-sleep

158. https://www.nhs.uk/live-well/sleep-and-tiredness/

159. https://theconversation.com/exercise-really-can-help-you-sleep-better-a
t-night-heres-why-that-may-be-192427

160. https://theconversation.com/exercise-really-can-help-you-sleep-better-a
t-night-heres-why-that-may-be-192427

161. https://link.springer.com/article/10.1007/s40279-018-1015-0

162. https://www.monash.edu/news/articles/natural-light-may-be-key-to-i
mproving-mood-and-reducing-insomnia2

163. https://www.sleephealthjournal.org/article/S2352-7218(18)30173-6/f
ulltext

164. https://www.cdc.gov/niosh/emres/longhourstraining/light.html

165. https://www.rcpsych.ac.uk/mental-health/problems-disorders/sleeping
-well

166. https://pubmed.ncbi.nlm.nih.gov/24720812/

167. https://www.rcpsych.ac.uk/mental-health/problems-disorders/sleeping
-well

168. https://thesleepcharity.org.uk/information-support/adults/sleep-hub/
sleep-meditation/

169. https://www.headspace.com/

170. https://www.ncbi.nlm.nih.gov/pmc/articles/PMC5426403/

171. https://www.ncbi.nlm.nih.gov/pmc/articles/PMC5426403/

172. https://medlineplus.gov/ency/patientinstructions/000951.htm

173. https://jamanetwork.com/journals/jamanetworkopen/fullarticle/275
2100

174. https://theconversation.com/positive-affirmations-how-talking-to-you
rself-can-let-the-light-in-199798

175. https://www.unisa.edu.au/media-centre/Releases/2020/when-youre-s
miling-the-whole-world-really-does-smile-with-you/

176. https://www.bmj.com/content/369/bmj.m2382

177. https://www.psychologytoday.com/gb/blog/where-science-meets-the-s
teps/201309/4-ways-sugar-could-be-harming-your-mental-health

178. https://joytripproject.com/finding-happiness-with-richard-davidson/

179. https://www.betterhealth.vic.gov.au/health/healthyliving/exercise-and
-mental-health

180. https://brighterworld.mcmaster.ca/articles/working-it-out-researchers-f
ind-exercise-may-help-seniors-fight-depression/

181. https://blog.smu.edu/research/2010/04/01/study-exercise-should-be
-prescribed-more-often-for-depression-anxiety/

182. https://www.mindtools.com/a5eygum/what-are-your-values

183. https://www.headspace.com/

184. https://www.wakingup.com/

185. https://www.mayoclinic.org/diseases-conditions/depression/expert-ans
wers/vitamin-b12-and-depression/faq-20058077

186. https://www.bu.edu/sph/news/articles/2022/sense-of-purpose-in-life
-may-be-linked-to-mortality-risk/

187. https://www.campaigntoendloneliness.org/threat-to-health/

188. https://www.nia.nih.gov/news/social-isolation-loneliness-older-people
-pose-health-risks

189. https://www.theguardian.com/science/2023/feb/22/exercise-and-satisf
ying-relationships-are-the-secrets-to-good-health-in-later-life

190. https://dailynews.mcmaster.ca/articles/on-international-day-of-older-p
ersons-mcmaster-experts-weigh-in-on-what-it-takes-to-age-well/

191. https://doi.org/10.1080/13607863.2022.2144130

192. https://news.osu.edu/why-some-friends-make-you-feel-more-supporte
d-than-others/

193. https://www.sciencedaily.com/releases/2014/08/140829135448.htm

194. https://www.cnn.com/2017/06/28/us/98-year-old-arrested-trnd/index.html

195. https://www.heart.org/en/news/2020/07/08/why-stay-in-touch-while-keeping-distant-its-only-human

196. https://www.plymouth.ac.uk/news/research-shows-that-people-overestimate-benefits-and-underestimate-risks-of-medical-interventions

197. https://www.england.nhs.uk/shared-decision-making/why-is-shared-decision-making-important/

198. https://www.healthinaging.org/medications-older-adults/medications-work-differently-older-adults

199. https://www.healthinaging.org/tools-and-tips/tip-sheet-ten-medications-older-adults-should-avoid-or-use-caution

200. https://www.healthinaging.org/tools-and-tips/tip-sheet-ten-medications-older-adults-should-avoid-or-use-caution

201. https://bjgp.org/content/early/2023/01/23/BJGP.2022.0181

202. https://www.healthinaging.org/medications-older-adults/medications-work-differently-older-adults

203. https://www.ncbi.nlm.nih.gov/books/NBK499956/

204. https://qualitysafety.bmj.com/content/30/2/96

205. https://www.singlecare.com/blog/news/medication-errors-statistics/

206. https://www.ncbi.nlm.nih.gov/pmc/articles/PMC539473/

207. https://www.cell.com/med/fulltext/S2666-6340(22)00173-8

208. https://www.thelancet.com/journals/lancet/article/PIIS0140-6736(22)01545-8/fulltext

209. https://www.nia.nih.gov/health/dietary-supplements-older-adults

210. https://www.dietaryguidelines.gov/sites/default/files/2021-03/Dietary_Guidelines_for_Americans-2020-2025.pdf

211. https://theconversation.com/vitamin-b12-deficiency-is-a-common-health-problem-that-can-have-serious-consequences-but-doctors-often-overlook-it-192714

212. https://www.escardio.org/The-ESC/Press-Office/Press-releases/Climb-stairs-to-live-longer

213. https://hr.duke.edu/wellness/exercise-fitness/take-stairs

214. https://www.jsams.org/article/S1440-2440(22)00083-4/fulltext

215. https://youtu.be/yNqCRm0jRbo

216. https://www.sciencedaily.com/releases/2023/03/230303175844.htm

217. https://www.sciencedaily.com/releases/2013/09/130905113711.htm

218. https://www.inc.com/melissa-chu/announcing-your-goals-makes-you-less-likely-to-ach.html

219. https://www.ucl.ac.uk/school-life-medical-sciences/news/2019/feb/making-goals-public-could-hinder-weight-loss

Printed in Great Britain
by Amazon